I SHOULD WAKE BEFORE I DIE

FIELD NOTES FROM THE VALLEY OF THE SHADOW (WITH SNACKS!)

ELISA L. EVERTS

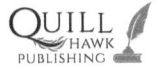

QUILL HAWK PUBLISHING

Cover design by Ava Wood, Fins and Feathers Designs

ISBN: 978-1-965142-76-9 (Paperback)

ISBN: 978-1-965142-77-6 (Hardback)

ISBN: 978-1-965142-54-7 (eBook)

Library of Congress Control Number: 2026900483

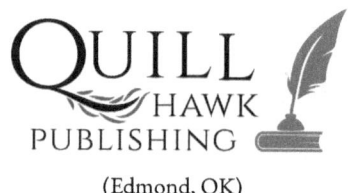

(Edmond, OK)

For Brian and Diane.

I couldn't save your lives, but I have tried to savor them all these years. And I will do my damnedest to make your light shine on others far beyond the grave.

"When my heart would explode,
She stepped in to reload.
And the floor gave way to a door. . ."

—Elisa L. Everts, *The Magical Sands of Time*

CONTENTS

PREFACE

Dear Reader

If you're holding this book, you have your own relationship with the Valley of the Shadow of Death.

Maybe you've already been through it. Maybe—God forbid—you're going through it now. Maybe you know someone who didn't make it out.

Before I say anything else, let me thank you for letting me sit with you in the dark, however briefly. Your pain is a holy place, and I will take my shoes off in the presence of your wound.

This book tells one story—mine. It's full of metaphors and zigzags, deep love and irreverent humor, quiet epiphanies and messy contradictions. It was born not from answers, but from questions, and from astonishment: that even in the shadow of death, light kept breaking through.

Let me be clear: I don't think everyone's grief should look like mine. This is not a how-to guide. It's a field report from one traveler to another. Healing isn't a straight line. My journey didn't end with these pages, and neither will yours.

I don't believe pain always transforms, or that sorrow flows neatly into meaning. Some losses remain unspeakably wrong.

My younger brother Brian died when I was four. My dearest friend Diane died decades later. Their deaths will never be okay. I will never be "at peace" with their deaths or their absence. And yet, their love is woven into every page of this book and into the fabric of my soul.

I'll be honest: if gallows humor isn't your companion, as it is mine, some of these pages might be uncomfortable. Humor is one way I manage adversity. It's how I whistle in the dark.

You might find moments here that feel too light, too hopeful, too poetic, or too raw. You might wonder why I joke about dying, or why I survived when someone you love didn't. You might wish I'd said more about this divine energy I'm comfortable calling *God*. Or less. I understand.

What I hope, above all, is that you don't have to make your journey through this valley alone. I've done that. It took me almost twenty years, and it really, really sucked.

I wish I'd had a book like this, or a soul like me, to bear witness to my agony. If something in these pages brings you any comfort or any light, if it speaks to you in your pain—then it has done what I hoped it would do.

With deep respect for your story, standing here with my shoes off and my heart open,

Elisa

INTRODUCTION

Just in Case You Don't Buy This Book

Just in case you don't buy this book, let me give you a gift. This is the most important thing I learned from cancer and grief: Life is not beautiful because it is long, my loves. It is beautiful because it is deep—full of love, full of joy, full of grace, and full of light. I just want to plant that seed in your mind, where I pray it will grow into a lovely flowering tree of hope, whether you read any further or not. If we don't turn our focus to making what life we have beautiful, it doesn't really matter how long we live.

I first wrote this book as a cancer memoir. But as it unfolded, I realized that I was writing about much more. This is a book about death, dying, and bereavement, about healing, meaning-making, and the strange, luminous beauty that can rise from the ashes of our losses. It's about learning to live deeply, to grieve fully, to love fiercely, and to wake up before we die.

Granted, cancer is one of the main characters; grief and death are the others. They raise their ugly heads as the primary antagonists in my story. Cancer, like death and grief, can be a bully. People often feel it is rubbing their faces in the dirt with a knee in their backs. You, however, are not some hapless, helpless hostage. You have so much agency and light for protecting yourself from their ravages.

I wanted to call this book *Stage Four? Hold My Beer: Cancer Is Not the Boss of Me*. (Though I decided that, one, it wasn't really about cancer, and two, it didn't quite have the loving, hopeful tone I was aiming for.) Still, my favorite comment shortly after my diagnosis with stage four pancreatic cancer was from my friend Mike, who said, "Elisa's all like, 'I have stage four cancer. Hold my beer.'"

If you're not familiar with that meme, there's usually some good ole boy like my brother being told he can't clear the barn with his muscle car. And he says, "Hold my beer," while he proceeds to race up a ramp and fly over the barn, presumably with the greatest of ease. I felt so affirmed and encouraged by Mike's comment that I really wanted to put it on the front of a T-shirt—or a book.

I am, however, so aware that cancer crashes into each life differently, into different places in one's biography, with different levels of horror, loss, and grace. I do not for a moment mean to make light of your cancer or that of your loved one. I am simply telling my story—how my cancer felt to me at the very particular (and fortunate) point where it fell into my life.

Where Does the Calm Come From?

The fact is, when I realized I did have a rather unusual calm about my terminal diagnosis, I began to explore the reasons for that calm. It turns out it had a lot to do with the fact that cancer was not my first rodeo.

I had spent years in the kind of choking grief that makes you wish you were dead yourself. I got very familiar with the terrain of the Valley of the Shadow of Death and the ghouls that lurk in its depths. But in the end, I am pleased to report: I did not make it my permanent address.

Mind you, I spent almost 20 years there—it was beginning to feel permanent. And when I tell you I know the terrain, I mean blindfolded with my hands tied behind my back. I didn't just visit the Valley; I pitched a tent, learned the language, mapped the underworld. But eventually I clawed my way out and emerged in the glorious light.

So, by the time the ER doctor told me I might have a year to live, my light was so bright it could not be so easily snuffed out. I felt grief, but at the same time, it did not steal my joy. And it didn't touch my peace. It wasn't denial. It was perspective.

I will tell you where that surprising calmness came from. I will also tell you about the times when I wanted to fling myself off a mountainside to get free of grief. And I will tell you about all the funny thoughts that floated through like sunlight filtering through the shade of trees and brought extra light to my path.

If I succeed, you will laugh, you will cry, you will kiss twenty bucks goodbye . . . and you will say hello to hope because this glimpse of light will have punched a hole in that black canopy of gloom and doom that has been threatening to extinguish your light.

You may feel like your light has just been blown out by an icy wind. Please do not be afraid. There is still light in your story. In fact, this darkness may make your light shine so much more brilliantly than it ever has. I'm going to show you the light in mine just in case you are having trouble seeing the light in yours.

Different Journeys

We have all made this trip to the present moment in bodies as unique as our journeys. Every body is as exquisitely unique as the (auto)biography it peoples. With each event, each thought, experience, and choice, we have each woven our own stories, embroidering our names and identities into the tapestries of our lives.

Knowing this, I would never claim to have blazed a trail for anyone in my own bumbling journey of cancer, grief, and inner healing. I do not know your path. I do not know the story of your heart or the story of your body (though I would love to). So, I ask myself: can I shed any light on your path, knowing that I have arrived at my place of healing and joy and hope by walking down another?

I only know how much light has been shed upon my path by the stories of other lives so different from my own. Perhaps light transcends sameness and identicality. That is my wish in offering my story to you, that you would find a transcendent light here as you walk through your own dark valley.

This Is Not a Book About How to Not Die

This is not a tale of my heroic fight for my life and how I vanquished illness through my amazing powers of positive thinking or the sheer will to live—although, hopefully, some of those elements are present. It's not a story about how I beat cancer in the usual sense, where "beating cancer" means definitely not getting dead.

It's not about my quest to *not* die. It's about how grief almost killed me earlier in my life, and how I ultimately overcame that grief and rose from the dead. After that, it came to be about my quest to live and love (and yes—please don't gag—definitely laugh) and to make my life as beautiful as I can, however much there is left.

This book is not a map for surviving cancer. If anything, it is a map to surviving grief. It's the map I used. You may find the terrain of your grief differs, and I honor that. The fact remains that when you successfully survive grief, if cancer or some other catastrophe comes, you'll be ready.

Moreover, cancer, grief, and death are not merely physical threats. Of course, they are physical. But they don't just happen to our bodies. They happen to our souls. And I think that if we do not tend to our souls as we tend to our bodies, it might be our undoing.

I am not talking about getting religious (although I honor those for whom that is a cherished path to spirituality). I am talking about being spiritual. What I mean is that I don't want to focus on laying out rules, but on nurturing your soul by demonstrating that the path through grief leads to spiritual growth and joy.

I believe that we can feed each other's souls by sharing our stories. And it is in that hopeful spirit that I share mine with you.

Critically, when we care for our souls, we also care for our bodies. For me, this means attending to my mind, my emotions, and my purpose—to how I am an expression of love in this world. I think our main spiritual work is to figure out who we are, why we are here, what we have to give and receive. And I think we must take charge of our stories to imbue our lives with the meaning we choose.

I decided cancer and death would not co-opt my story. They would not be the boss of me. They would not hog center stage. They would not distract me from the purpose of my life (which I feel is finding expressions of love that are uniquely mine) by making me turn all my attention on myself and my illness.

The purpose of life is not mere self-preservation. That's tautology. It means you exist to exist. It's futility.

More Than One Way to Win the Fight Against Cancer

There's more than one way to win the fight against cancer and death. I reject the standard narrative that suggests that if my life does come to an early end, that means I "lost" the fight. I can win the fight by how I spend my life and how lovingly, beautifully, powerfully, deliberately I live each moment.

I can win the fight by simply taking control of my own story. When cancer and death get their way, they write a horror story. Unfortunately, that is precisely what they did to me for more than twenty years. But I don't like horror stories (sorry, Stephen King—it's nothing personal). I like beautiful stories full of love and redemption.

By the time I healed from my personal horror stories and a terminal cancer diagnosis threatened to suck me into yet another one, I decided I would write a beautiful story with the last chapter of my life—writing defiantly around cancer and death but not elevating them beyond their due.

You'll no doubt want to know how I reached a state of being in the world where cancer was not such a big deal. The fact is, I had already spent a very long time in hell battling many demons, each of which was, in itself, a formidable foe. And I have to tell you, they almost destroyed me.

But I found my resurrection power and climbed out of hell. And by the time I did, cancer and death could no longer scare me.

May These Pages Feed You

When I was given my grim diagnosis, I started a blog—essentially a love letter to my nearest and dearest—in which I hoped to help them grieve and to see the beauty of their lives. Since I've been down this dark and treacherous road through the Valley of the Shadow of Death more than once, I thought perhaps I could light some lamps for them along the way.

That blog evolved into this book. I have made very few changes to the blog posts here, but I have rearranged them and added a fair amount of other material I felt would be helpful to you, my new readers (and welcome!).

As a result, you will find a whole choir of voices among these chapters—all of them mine. This book is a prism, and each chapter refracts the same light through a different lens—scholar, daughter, believer, skeptic, joker, mourner, survivor.

I did not even try to write with one voice. I tried to write with my whole self, since making our selves whole is, after all, the point.

If you picked up this book, you are probably very weary. Your soul needs nourishment for this journey. You probably don't need religion just now. You need spiritual food—something nourishing, tender, and true.

Our stories are one of our richest sources of spiritual nourishment I know of, and in that spirit, I offer mine.

I'll admit, part of my story is going to feel more like chemotherapy than enjoying your favorite meal. But I promise that at the end of this story, there is resurrection and new life and a strength that made stage IV cancer and the threat of death virtually bow before me.

I know that sounds arrogant. I'm just trying to say that I didn't let them tower over me, all menacing and ominous. I stood as the victor after having spent so many years as a victim.

It doesn't matter what your faith flavor is. Your soul needs nourishment. I find this kind of nourishment to be very good for your eyes. It enables us to see our lives in a new way.

If you will let me, I would love to feed your soul from these pages. I would love to feed you laughter—but also healing tears. I would love to feed you meaning and beauty. I would love to feed you the kind of hope that is valid whether you live or die and is not necessarily dependent on a belief in an afterlife.

I would love to feed you resurrection.

A Map for the Reader

This book unfolds like a soul's migration: downward first, into the valley where everything once known is stripped bare. There, in the stillness, I learn from grief, and unknowing begins its quiet work. Then comes the slow turning—toward meaning, beauty, and a language large enough to hold both sorrow and joy. Finally, the ascent: not back to what was, but into a life made joyful and beautiful by love, redefined by presence. These pages are a map of that journey, but they are also an invitation—to wake before you die, to live while you are still here, and to trust that even in shadow, the light is already waiting.

— • —

PART I: AND SO IT BEGINS

1

ONE KEY TO THEM ALL

I hate to be the one to point this out, but before you can get to resurrection, you have to die.

If you have ever grieved deeply, you've already done that. Because when grief guts you, it feels like a death.

And not just the death of the person you lost. It's the death of the self you were when they were still here. It's the death of certainty, of identity, of the world you thought you lived in.

A terminal diagnosis can feel like that, too.

What Is the Greatest Grief?

I died twice before I ever faced my own impending death—once when my brother Brian died in childhood, and once when my friend Diane died far too young.

After a very, very long grief, I finally reached a beautiful state of healing. So, when they told me I would die too, I was relatively unfazed. They told me I might live a year, with treatment. I was shocked—but I wasn't afraid.

Because I had already died and been spiritually and emotionally resurrected, I had an amazing peace and calm about my early physical demise. I started making plans to make it as beautiful a final chapter as I possibly could.

Many would say that grieving your own death is the greatest grief. And yes, I think that's true—but mostly because when you face the loss of your own life, you also face the loss of everyone and everything you love. It is the ultimate letting go.

You don't just lose yourself. You lose everyone, all at once.

Some people might argue that all grief is ultimately for the self. And maybe that's true. But I know this: when I faced the possibility of my own death, it didn't feel like I was grieving me. It felt like I was grieving everyone I would have to leave behind. What is life, if not the totality of our relationships? All the beautiful people we love—and who love us?

The Grief That Nearly Killed Me

These griefs are colossal. But for me, the greatest grief I've known wasn't for myself or for the people I would lose. The greatest grief was the one I felt responsible for: the death of my baby brother.

That grief wasn't just loss—it was soul-crushing guilt. A burden I carried alone for years.

I never would have imagined that my brother's death would have anything to do with my cancer. But it turns out that resolving that early childhood grief was essential to facing my terminal diagnosis.

There was no kick-ass energy to face cancer—or anything else—until that mother wound was healed.

Diana Gabaldon writes in *An Echo in the Bone*: "All loss is one, and one loss becomes all, a single death the key to the gate that bars memory."[1] That turned out to be hauntingly true in my own life, though it took me almost forty years to figure it out.

Understanding what happened with my brother Brian was the key to understanding how I processed every other loss.

I Should Wake Before I Die

That cultural reference in the subheading might (fortunately?) be lost on younger readers. There used to be a common childhood prayer that included the line: "If I should die before I wake, I pray the Lord my soul to take"—no doubt emerging from a time when child mortality was an ever-present reality. I think that line has been softened in more contemporary versions.

But I'll tell you what troubles me more than dying in your sleep: never waking before you die. Most people, as a therapist friend once said to me, go to their graves without ever getting their deepest wounds healed. And what a tragedy that is.

Life is so much more beautiful when you are healed.

Facing a terminal diagnosis is not for wimps. It takes a considerable degree of emotional health. If you have unresolved grief in your life, a cancer diagnosis is going to be infinitely harder to cope with than if you have faced and integrated your past pain.

If you have grief hidden in your bones and buried deep in your soul, I fear that cancer—or some other crisis—may rip you open the way my beloved friend Diane's death ripped open the wound of my unresolved childhood grief. I'll share more about that in the coming chapters.

But if I could help you ward off such a fate—that would be one of my dearest wishes.

Thank God I Woke

Thank God, I woke before I died.

If I die today or next month or next year, it will not be a great tragedy. Fifty-eight is, after all, more than half a pencil (see Chapter Twenty-Four for this hysterical allusion).

The key discovery is this: I have reached a place of great happiness and contentment.

I had to go through hell to get here. But I got my wounds healed. I found all kinds of redemption before my life came to completion. Everything else is a bonus. I am now just reveling in a bounty of grace.

And I wish the same bounty of grace for all of you.

I hope that by telling my story, some of you might see parallels that help you, too—get to healing. And from there, to that grace.

Timeline

Here is a quick timeline of my life in case my nonlinear narrative style gives you whiplash.

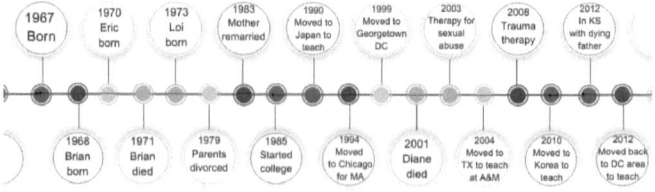

---

1. Gabaldon, Diana. *An Echo in the Bone*. Delacorte Press, 2009.

2

Who Is Writing Our Stories?

Our Very Different Journeys

Before I begin my story, let me ask you, how did you come to this moment where you are now reading this sentence I have written for you, hoping that you would? I am sure you have come by a very different path than the one by which I arrived.

How did you manage your journey from birth to this moment? Did you determine your exact destination before you departed? Did you carefully plan your trip with compass and map in hand? Did you stick to the plan and never veer off, distracted by things you saw along the way? Did you buy all the right equipment and dress appropriately? Did you train your body for the rugged terrain before you set off?

Did you plan healthy meals and manage to procure them? Did you never stumble or injure yourself? Did you pack a first aid kit that had everything you needed? Did you have a helpful traveling companion? Did you remember to enjoy your journey, stopping to play and to savor the beauty of each new place that each day, each series of steps on your path brought you?

If you did, I bow to you. Please write a book for me, too. I think I hoped to manage the journey of my life like that. But I rather feel that I have stumbled along more often than not, sometimes bleakly, sometimes more blithely and blissfully, sometimes feeling bloody and bludgeoned by pain and calamity, and often so blindly, to the crossroads of this moment where our minds meet now.

Are You Writing Your Life or Is It Writing You?

I think there may have been a time when I was very young that I thought that I would write my life. But eventually, I began to wonder whether my life was writing me. Did you ever think this? Once I thought that I could choose the setting, plot, and characters and choose my own happy ending and write a beautiful final chapter at the end of a very, very long book.

(Now please do not get your undies in a wad that I am about to use the word *God*. There is something I am comfortable calling *divine*—that life spark that fuels and animates us. Call it *The Universe, The Great Spirit,* or *The Force.* Maybe *Energy* or *Source* or *Life* or even the *Collective Consciousness.* Call it *Bob.* Or *Matilda.* Whatever it is that is the source of love and grace and art and inspiration.)

Actually, I thought that God and I would write this book together. In fact, I suppose I thought that She would be the primary author and I just someone who wrote it *with* Her. That I could tag along in the backseat and just plead like a child that She choose desirable destinations. That was prayer. And my role was passive.

Some of us, when we were younger, especially if we are Americans, thought that we could write our own lives, that we could determine our own destinies.

Americans love to quote the poet William Ernest Henley (usually without knowing some critical context such as that he wrote it from his hospital bed after having lost a leg to tuberculosis), in declaring passionately, "I am the master of my fate!"[1] Others of us have always felt that we were characters in a story we did not write.

Sometimes we believe that a terrible God wrote that story. Sometimes we believe that it was written by our parents or other major characters who stormed through our lives, manipulating situations, creating emotional environments we may or may not have even been able to breathe through, acting upon us.

Some perceive themselves as warriors and others, victims. I wonder how many people actually feel that they are writing their lives themselves and how long it takes before something happens to them that convinces them otherwise. Like cancer, for instance. Nobody is going to write cancer into their story (unless they are very mentally ill), and then I'm pretty sure they would write it right back out.

It is such a glorious gift that, as human beings, we do have the power to choose. But we do not have an unlimited set of choices before us. There are so many people and events and features that force their way into our lives, and we have no control over them. These we do not choose.

In my youth, I bemoaned that I was a character born into a crap story. A mentally ill father who was unemployed for most of my childhood, a blind mother, poverty and social stigma, partial deafness, sexual abuse, the tragic death of my baby brother and its attendant trauma, betrayal, abandonment, grief, suicidality, unemployment, singleness, childlessness, complex PTSD and . . . cancer (and trust me, that is not even a complete inventory!) ... these were frankly not story elements I would have chosen for myself.

Also, I would have given myself a different nose and probably taken a pass on the chicken lips (seriously, when the Everts smile, our lips disappear). I would have also supplied myself with a butt (I do not know what She was thinking? A casual glance at my person and you will realize it's not like she ran out of cellulite!).

Fairy Tale Life

No, I would have written a fairy tale. Well, I would have written the second half of the fairy tale. Actually, who am I kidding? I'd have written just the last bit—I would have skipped the first ninety percent with all the "adventure" and gone straight to the happy ending. (Here I can't help but imagine Prince Humperdink in *The Princess Bride* urging the eloquent clergyman, "SKIP to the end!"[2]) Have you ever noticed that when we say someone has led a *fairy tale life*, we are thinking of the happy ending? In fact, most fairy tales have very Grimm (hee hee) complicating actions leading up to those happy endings. We forget that bit.

When we say, *"He lived a fairy tale life,"* we almost certainly do not mean he spent twenty years of it as a frog. We mean, of course, that he lived as a prince.

But if he was born a prince and lived as a prince his whole life—well, that's not a very interesting story. I wouldn't pay money for that book, would you? Not unless he slew dragons blindfolded with his hands tied behind his back while playing the harmonica, or built a hanging garden on the moon, say.

Generally, we prefer rags-to-riches stories over look-how-Richy-got-richer stories. We love tales where the underdog defies the odds and rises from ignominy to glory.

For other people, anyway. Maybe not for ourselves.

Yet complications are the stuff of great stories. So are villains. The best stories have the most conflict and the worst villains. And cancer is a truly evil villain. Ok, I'm beginning to realize that maybe I should send the universe a check for creating characters and complications that make my story such potentially compelling reading. Thank you, Universe, for making my life so interesting. Nothing bores me faster than a paint-by-numbers plot and characters with the depth of a pancake.

But the point I'm trying to make is that for so many years, I was just a character in my own story. I didn't see how I could possibly be the narrator of all these objectionable nonoptional story elements. I was a beleaguered character; I wasn't even a heroine. I was someone stuff happened to. I wasn't someone who made stuff happen. And I certainly didn't happen to stuff.

When a writer sets her pen to page, she has, theoretically, the whole world of words and ideas to choose from in creating the book before her. And she can write anything she wishes: a romance, a textbook, a fantasy, a horror story, an epic poem, an account of fact or fiction. And, oh! Most importantly, she can edit the hell out of that book! She can even scrap it and start a brand-new book.

Collaborative Culinary Throwdown

Our lives are not quite like this. They are more like a culinary throwdown between chefs who are given a set of ingredients they did not choose and asked to make a delicious dish of these (and sometimes there is a discrete time limit). In that case, as in too many lives, we feel that the dish must be judged delicious by someone else.

But what I want to ask you is: how does it taste *to you*? Is this the meal you wanted to eat, or the one you thought would win the most applause? Are you savoring your own life, or just serving it up for approval? And what role did loving the same meals play in choosing the people you love? This is the same choice grief offers us, too: to live according to someone else's expectations, or to shape a life that feels true to our own soul.

This brings me back to the wisdom of Glennon Doyle: "Do not disappoint yourself."[3] Basically, she says, "Stop worrying about disappointing everyone else, and consider in what ways you are disappointing yourself. And stop."

How can we take the ingredients before us and create a meal that sates us, that nourishes all the needs of our bodies, and at the same time tickles and tantalizes our taste buds? Isn't it also true that our loved ones, the ones we choose to surround ourselves with, will find this dish delicious, too?

We don't get to choose all the ingredients of our stories. But we get to choose what we do with the ingredients we have.

Or perhaps we might think of it as a game of chess. The universe makes a move (a wonderful lover, cancer, a gift for music, a learning disability, etc.), and we make our move. We choose our response. Thus, writing our stories is kind of an interactive experience, which can actually be both more challenging and more fun than being in control of all the story elements.

At some point, I came to realize that I could tell my story differently. That I am not a mere character in my story; I am the heroine, but I am also the narrator. I get to choose my response to the people and events that come through my life, and I also get to decide what each part of my story means. Nobody else gets to define who I am or assign the meaning and cause/effect relationships of what has happened to me. Only I have that right. I own my story.

The stories we tell don't have to be grand. They can be whispered. Fragmented. Scribbled in the margins. What matters is that they move us toward agency—toward reclaiming some small measure of power, meaning, or voice in a world that can feel brutally out of control. Whether your story is a screaming anthem or a shaky note passed in class, it matters. Telling it can be a form of self-rescue. A way of saying, *This is mine. I get to say what it meant. I get to say how it ends.*

I have come to believe that I do indeed have the option—even the calling to be a co-author with the universe in writing my life. This requires creativity (which, by the way, I find to be a major depression buster that brings joy and beauty into my life), and creativity flows from the divine. She has imparted it to me as my birthright, and She does not expect me to use it to buy a cold bowl of soup. She expects my creative, collaborative authorship to bring me (and others!) joy.

Luckily, I figured this out before I got cancer because that perspective empowered me to take my story back from cancer before she could take me down a path even darker than the one I did travel.

Harvesting Light and Self-Fulfilling Prophecies

A few years before cancer, a poem came to me from the universe that has been feeding me ever since.

In the secret garden of my heart
I am growing . . .
Light!
Fueled by the flaming Spirit of God
that burns within my soul,
like a burning bush that does not expire
I am growing here a crop of fire!

As I began to tell myself this story, it became a self-fulfilling prophecy (I always think the best kind of prophesies are those that fulfill your self!). I discovered that I really could grow light in the secret garden of my heart, and I am so glad I did. And it turns out that light is a magical crop that begins to multiply itself. The more I shined on others, the more light grew inside me. I filled up my spiritual barns with light, bales of light stacked to the rafters. And I am so grateful that I did because I needed it for the long dark night of the soul I didn't see coming.

---

1. Henley, William Ernest. *Invictus*. 1875. *The Oxford Book of English Verse*, edited by Arthur Quiller-Couch, Oxford UP, 1919.

2. *The Princess Bride*. Directed by Rob Reiner, screenplay by William Goldman, performance by Cary Elwes, 20th Century Fox, 1987.

3. Doyle, Glennon. *Untamed*. The Dial Press, 2020

3

—•—

SMACKED UPSIDE THE HEAD WITH A CANCER STICK

Blind Date with the Grim Reaper

How many times has this happened to you? You're tooling down the highway of life, just minding your own damned business, when some monstrosity from hell emerges out of nowhere and smacks you upside the head?

Bruce Feiler (as I learned via Saleema Vellani[1]) calls these lifequakes.[2] I am now trying to decide whether a deathquake is the ultimate lifequake.

In the spring of 2020, there was so much joy and love flowing in, out, around, and through me. I had finally come to love myself and my life. I had gone from measuring my "happiness" level by how far below zero I was (-3 was begging God to take my life, -4 was actively planning my suicide—I never reached level -4, but I spent many years at -3), to being a 9 or a 10 almost all the time.

I was spiritually, emotionally, socially, physically, and professionally in the best, most hopeful season of my life in twenty years. I had risen from the dead. I was so excited about my new incipient career in speaking and writing. My life was a miracle I was eager to share with the world.

So, there I was, racing down the path to realizing my dreams, when suddenly the sky turned black, and my path took a twisty turn straight into a nightmare.

On May 22, 2020, the ER doctor basically set me up on a blind date with the Grim Reaper. He looked at me with way too much compassion and said, "You have stage four pancreatic cancer. You have tumors from your pancreas to your pelvis. Without treatment, you'll be dead in a matter of months."

I, in turn, looked at him like he had just stumbled out of a crack den. *Nobody in my family gets cancer! I am immune! Did you not get the memo??*

I was flabbergasted. Blew my head right off my shoulders. I couldn't have been more surprised if my parents had suddenly revealed I'd been adopted from an orphanage in Uganda (I am a pasty white girl from Kansas).

My mind spun like a roulette wheel. But when it stopped spinning, it came to rest on the year 2001, when I had cared for my dear friend Diane as she died of stomach cancer. For me, Diane's death was both sacred and scarring—horrific, but also holy. Deeply dark but punctuated with the brightest of lights. Nevertheless, the trauma of that experience left me so broken I could barely function. I cried heavily for seven years. She had just turned thirty.

She was in hard-core denial right up till a few weeks before she died. So much was left unsaid, undone, untended. I reflected on that extensively.

I Just Remembered I Have a Script for This

Even though I never expected to get cancer, after watching Diane suffer, I'd had many conversations with myself about what I would do—just hypothetically—if I were ever diagnosed with a really bad cancer.

Diane had one surgery, chemotherapy, and two more surgeries. She got a massive infection, and her wound would not close. She could not eat for the rest of her short life. For the sixty days it took her to die, all she could consume was ruby red grapefruit juice because that's the only thing that wouldn't clog her nasal-gastro tube, which she also had for the remaining sixty days of her life.

It was pure hell.

I wasn't doing that. I thought, *If I'm going to die swiftly, let's do palliative care and let me enjoy my people for whatever time I have left.*

So, as I sat there in the ER, I realized I'd had twenty years to think about it and concluded, *I know how to do this.* And I started calmly planning my final chapter from my hospital bed.

I don't think I started crying until they took me for the MRI. The tech told me to think of happy things, so I pictured the faces of my loved ones one by one.

Tears streamed down the sides of my face.

I know the choking, gut-wrenching, throat-squeezing devastation of grief. I knew how this was going to crush them. Each face made me dissolve into tears of grief, and I started sobbing in the machine. It was so hard to stop crying long enough to hold still for the imaging.

Happy thoughts? I thought of my very beloved cat (which, granted, would have been more appropriate when I was having the CAT scan earlier—or even the PET scan later). Even when I focused on her, I sobbed. All these years I'd been worried about how long she would live, and now it seemed she would outlive me.

I thought, *She will never understand why I disappeared.* The tears just kept streaming, and snot was making it damn near impossible to breathe.

When they slid me back out, the tech actually asked me, "Why are you sad?" I looked at her quizzically thinking, *Really? I don't think anybody goes in there expecting to find buried treasure in the recesses of her person!*

Cancer Is Not the Boss of Me

My life has been really messy, with more than the usual allotment of agony—but also perhaps more than the usual allotment of beauty. But messy. Not the work of art I wanted it to be.

I believe the point of me is to love people, and when I do that, joy flows out of me. I am pretty content that I have done this since childhood, but I had wanted to pour out so much more love with my life. And now it was coming to a rapid end.

You may have noticed that I am still alive to write this. There are some plot twists ahead, but no spoilers.

We do not get to choose the number of our days. We can only choose what we do with each day we are given. When you are diagnosed with a fatal disease, you feel like you have lost all control. I recognized I could not control my cancer, but I was also not going to let it control me.

Cancer is not the boss of me.

Just because I can't control everything does not mean I cannot control anything. There are many things I can control. I have many choices to make. I might not be able to control all the whats or the whens, but I have a lot to say about the hows.

Before my diagnosis, I had all these grand plans for pouring love into the world in the decades before me. When I found out my number was up, I felt like I was sitting in the audience planning my act for next week, when suddenly I was called on stage.

This is it! Next week is not going to happen. This is your last chance to shine. You have to give it all. You have to improvise and put everything you've got into this last dance.

This sense of destiny and purpose overwhelmed any potential sense of doom.

I love this quote from Marc Chagall: "Art must be an expression of love, or it is nothing." And Vincent van Gogh expressed what I consider the corollary: "I think there is nothing more artistic than loving people."

With those thoughts in my heart, I determined that if this was my last chapter, I would do my damnedest to go out in a blaze of beauty and to make my dying a work of art—my last act of love.

After three days, I did what writers do when anything remotely interesting happens to them—I started a blog.

The blog had more significance for me than it might have if I were not single and living alone in the time of the COVID pandemic lockdowns. I couldn't see anyone. I couldn't hug anyone. I didn't even have my cat with me.

So, the blog became the best place (besides Facebook, which was also a real lifeline) for me to communicate with everyone about my well-being, as well as to try to help them process what was happening to me. Like me, it was passionate and quirky and ranged from the silly to the sublime—and much of it has formed the backbone of this book.

There Are No Shortcuts, But Some Maps Are Better Than Others

Just in case you're having a sinking feeling that I might be one of those delusional positive thinkers whose rose-colored Ray-Bans filter out all the truly awful suffering of life, let me assure you: I know the soul-splitting agony of grief that can lay waste to your life for years.

I estimate that I have spent ten years of my life weeping. Three individual, noncontiguous years—and then seven years straight. During those years, I woke up crying, sometimes cried throughout the day, and when I got home from work, I cried myself to sleep.

Indeed, I cried in my sleep, a fact which fascinated my psychiatrists as much as it distressed my roommates.

I had Kleenex by the bed, in the car, on my desk. I am so good at crying that I can cry out of just one eye if I don't want the person on the other side of me (in church, for example) to see my tears.

I'm telling you this because I want you to understand that I am fully aware of the need to grieve and feel all the agony first. And I want you to know that my joy on this cancer journey has never been something I manufactured out of denial.

You cannot skip the pain of grief. You can't get through grief unless you first let yourself feel all of the pain, all of the feelings.

As Robert Frost famously wrote, "The best way out is always through."[3]

There are no shortcuts to healing. You don't get to skip the grief and jump straight to joy.

But in my case, I had already been grieving—for decades.

I had lost my baby brother as a child and my dearest friend Diane as an adult. Their deaths shattered me, and over time, I let most of the sorrow move through me. I had gushed grief (and gushed, and gushed, and gushed) until it was all washed out of me. I had cried my soul inside out.

In a way, I had pre-grieved. As Diana Gabaldon wrote that one death was the key to them all, Dylan Thomas also wrote, "After the first death, there is no other."[4]

That has been true for me.

The deepest grief had already carved a deep canyon in my soul, and I had already climbed out of it by the time of my diagnosis. I had reached an astonishing level of healing and happiness before I got cancer.

I'll tell you more about this in the chapters ahead.

My road to lifelong healing was long indeed. I wandered around in my (be)wilderness for nearly fifty years (1971–2019) before I found my healing spring.

There might not be any shortcuts to healing, but I'm pretty sure there is a more direct route.

What follows is the map I built—slowly, painfully, over time. It's not the map. It's my map. Your grief may look nothing like mine, and I honor that.

Still, if your path winds long and lonely, my hope is that something here might help you find your way a little sooner—or at least feel a little less lost while you're in the wilderness.

---

1. Vellani, Saleema. *Innovation Starts With I: Increase Your Influence. Ignite Your Impact.* Ripple Impact Publishing, 2024.

2. Feiler, Bruce. *Life Is in the Transitions: Mastering Change at Any Age*. William Morrow, 2023.

3. Frost, Robert. *A Servant to Servants*. In *North of Boston*, Henry Holt and Company, 1914.

4. Thomas, Dylan. *Collected Poems: 1934–1952*. New Directions, 1952.

4

Your Number Is Up

How long have you always imagined living? Are you one of those Peter Pans who never wanted to get old? Or are you one of those people who wants to break the world record for longevity?

Either way, have you always had some number in the back of your mind, some age you've always assumed you'd live to?

Based on my grandmother and great aunt's ages, I always kind of vaguely assumed that my number was in the late nineties. Finding out how low that number might actually be (by getting a grim diagnosis) will knock the wind right out of you.

Fortunately, I had given that prospect a lot of thought (even though I had assumed those musings to be strictly theoretical), so I was able to catch my breath with surprising alacrity.

The Blog: Loving Life to the Very Last Drop

On May 25, 2020, three days after my diagnosis, I started a blog I named *Loving Life to the Very Last Drop* with this introductory description (and the following introductory post):

When people find out their last chapter is going to be shorter and show up sooner than they had planned for, they say they're dying. I'm not dying. I'm living. Right up to the very last moment. I invite you to join me on this journey for as long as you dare. It is not for the faint of heart, but it is a sacred experience like no other. I think it's possible to grieve joyfully. Let's find out if I'm right.

Your Number Is Up

Monday, May 25, 2020

I did not expect the number to be 53.

Which is what I turned on April 24, 2020.

Three days ago, I got the ticket.

I went to the ER expecting maybe gallstones... and learned, to my astonishment, that I had advanced pancreatic cancer.

There is almost no cancer in my family. I really always believed I was off Scot-free. We had longevity in our veins! Multiple nonagenarians! By my generation, I figured we'd be pushing 120.

I had such plans! They were amazing, beautiful, totally achievable plans—and I was making great strides toward them.

I was, to say the least, nonplussed.

At the advent of my fifty-first birthday, just two years prior, I had written this:

Over the Hill

I think at 51
I am probably officially
considered over the hill.
I mean, I guess that assumes the
hill is the midpoint of my life
and we know I'm only
going to live to 100, right?
Perish the thought!
I like to think that hill
is closer to 70.

"It's all downhill from here,"
they'll say.
And what does that mean?
It's easier the rest of the way?
After all this grueling work to
get to the "top," you can
now slide down the opposite side
in relative ease?

Or does it mean it's all
a decline from here?
Nothing to look forward to,
just winding up your life
and looking back fondly
on all those reckless,
raucous days of your youth?
Mine so disappointingly misspent
on all that needless goodytwoshoery . . .

Or is it more of a physical metaphor?
After the painfully slow rise,
the ball will now rush down to the bottom,
plummeting me to the depths of my demise
in what will feel like mere seconds
with the deftness of a roller coaster?
Am I now rolling toward my
death at an accelerated speed?

My God, did I put one toe in my grave today?!

I think not.
The trajectory of my life is not a broken line
with the point of a hill in the middle,
hanging a sharp right to the grave.

I see the trajectory of my life as a single line
that rises from the earth to the horizon,
into the sky, as far as the eye can see
–indeed, beyond what the eye can see!

My trajectory is like what the psalmist describes,
declaring that the path of a beautiful soul
is like the light of dawn
that grows brighter and brighter
until the full day!

I'm not over the hill.

There is no hill.

Well, I clearly didn't expect *this*.
But I stand by my poem.
Life is beautiful, and I will continue savoring it as I have finally learned to do in the penultimate chapter of my life.
And when I come to the last page of my final chapter, I am not going to write *The End*. That's just so negative! I think I'm going to write *The Completion*.
Getting to the last page is reaching the zenith of this stage of the soul's journey. It's growing brighter and brighter until the full day.
I want to make sure I write this final chapter as beautifully as I may.
Stay tuned to find out whether I succeed.
Later that week, I posted something I had written in 2018—little guessing I was establishing myself as a minor prophet (it is appropriate to politely chortle here).

The Number of My Days

Friday, May 29, 2020

When I was 40, much like when I was 5,
I felt like I could spend days forever and never run out.
I was rich with days.
I burned through them like newspapers on the fire.

After I turned 50, I finally understood
that my days were actually countable.
And their number is finite.

When I spend one, like a candle
Yielding its wax to fire and time,
There is no reconstitution.
Nothing left but a simple pool of wax like the
lingering memories of the day.
Or some days, like some candles, the wax just
burns away with the fire, leaving nothing in its wake.

I thought of God, doling out the days like
She doles out oxygen– in seemingly endless quantities,
I could never breathe it all up.

But after I was 50,
I began to understand the psalmist, who
(too candidly for my taste)
laments (but not without wonder)
how God knows the exact number of our days.
And each one has a price, a cost, a value.

Each one a canvas in the private exhibit of my life.
Will I paint something memorable, something memory-worthy?
Or will I leave it blank,
or merely covered with a background of gray?

Will I throw it away the way I breathe out
my seemingly inexhaustible supply of oxygen?

Will I heedlessly feed each canvas to the fire–
lost works of art that never were,
that never became because I never realized
I would be leaving dark, ugly holes
on the walls of my memory by not painting them?

When I am 80, I suspect I will feel all the more keenly–
but in my 50's, I already understand
that each day is a precious gem given to me–
uncut, rough and raw, ready to be cut
into exquisite gleaming works of artistry,
magic stones that carry within little fires of their own.
Or will they be thrown away like pearls to the swine,
like grass to the fire, like dust to the wind?

Oh, the pearls and diamonds I have lost
by not being awake to the number of my days!

By the time I penned these words, I had lost two brothers, my father, four grandparents, and one unspeakably dear friend—among others.

They ranged in age from three to ninety-five.

There is just no telling what your number will be.

The First Time I Thought My Number Was Up
Wednesday, May 27, 2020

I remember this so clearly, even though it happened more than fifty years ago, in 1972. I was five. It was the year after my brother died, on a hot summer's day in upstate New York, at my aunt's pool.

I ran around on the sandpapery hot cement, marveling at how even the water that splashed onto it was hot under my tender feet. I reveled in the smell of chlorine—the smell of summer, the smell of play, the smell of joy.

My parents sat languidly by the pool, half-asleep. My mother, being blind, left it to my father to keep an eye on me since I couldn't swim yet.

I walked over to the edge of the shallow end and sat down, kicking my feet in the water. I laughed as the cold water splashed up on me, but the hot cement was burning my bottom. So I slid, gasping, into the pool and stood by the side, where I could hang on, my feet just touching the slippery cement floor.

Oh, so curious, I maneuvered myself along the wall of the pool until I reached the floating rope that separated the shallow end from the deep. I edged out toward that precarious line, convinced I was safe because I was holding onto the rope. I could feel with my toes the precise spot where the floor dropped off—a slippery corner that sloped suddenly toward the deep end.

Naturally, with my toes, I flirted with that corner. Then, in a flash of wild pre-kindergarten rebellion, I stuck just the tip of my toe over the edge into the deep.

Much to my surprise, I lost my balance and tumbled down that slope, under the water.

I flailed my arms and legs but couldn't reach the surface. My eyes were wide open. I remember how the light shone through the waves, showing up like bright fragments of glass on the blue walls and the white floor of the pool. Water was getting in my nose. It stung.

And now I could taste the chlorine.

I was still flailing, but not so vigorously now. And I just thought, very calmly, *Huh. I guess I'm going to die.*

It made sense. Brian had just died last year. It must be my turn. And I had a very strange kind of stoic peace about it. *This is happening. I am drowning.*

I didn't feel afraid. I just felt resigned.

And just as I was preparing to leave this world, I felt an enormous splash next to me. My father had jumped in and he popped me up out of the water, splashing and sputtering, looking like a little drowned rat—but very much alive.

He wrapped me in a towel and sat me down on the edge of a lounge chair. I sat there shivering and thinking, *Huh. I guess it wasn't my turn after all.*

Reflection

I'm not sure how old I was when I stopped thinking I might die at any time, but I never lost my awareness of the brevity and uncertainty of life.

On the other hand, I've always taken most adversity and setbacks in relative stride since that fateful day in 1971 when I lost my brother. Anything less than being physically present and involved in the event that took someone's life seemed to me relatively small potatoes.

I did a lot of silent emotional hemorrhaging about that loss, but I was not easily riled by most of what life threw at me—even as I waited, always, for the other shoe to drop.

5

HIDE AND WATCH

My Extraordinary Education

Shortly after my diagnosis of terminal cancer, several of my closest friends said something along the lines of, "I don't think I would be handling it with so much grace."

Grace? I hardly felt I was making a ballet out of things.

But it *is* true that I was surprisingly calm about it all. A few people even asked me where my strength came from. The question made me curious myself, and it led me to reflect deeply on the reasons for my equanimity.

Let me assure you: this peace (as I've written elsewhere about grace) didn't come floating out of my person like rainbows from the nether regions of a unicorn. On reflection, I realized I had built this fortress—brick by brick—from the rubble of my war-torn life.

Simply put, stage four cancer was not my first rodeo.

It wasn't even my worst.

It barely makes the top five—and that would still be true even if I were already dead from it.

I realize not everyone is lucky enough to get into the school of hard knocks, and I don't want to brag, but I got a full ride.

To be honest, I think maybe I was a legacy student, too.

As I mentioned earlier, I was the firstborn child of a blind mother and a mentally ill father (untreated bipolar disorder), with a considerable degree of poverty and dysfunction in the mix. We lived in thirteen different places by the time I was nine. I went to five different elementary schools. For much of that time, we lived far below the welfare class. Again and again, we found ourselves just an onion skin away from homeless.

At twelve, I had a benign brain tumor removed and underwent major reconstructive surgery on my ear. I'm still deaf in that ear (which, as I'll explain later, may have indirectly caused my brother's death). I was abused by several different men, yada yada—you get the picture. There was stuff.

But as I reflect, I would say that the very worst thing that ever happened to me was my brother's death.

When I was four and my brother was three, he was hit and killed by a tractor-trailer. I was supposed to have his hand.

But I didn't.

And I had no idea how profoundly devastating this was to my baby soul until I was forty-one years old. I spent nearly forty years wandering in the wilderness of unresolved grief.

I'll tell you more about that when I tell you about the aftermath of my dear friend's death because I didn't realize I was still hemorrhaging from that childhood wound until I found myself grieving *hard* for my friend—*seven years* after she died—and it finally occurred to me that this might not be normal.

(Go ahead and roll your eyes. It's funny in a macabre sort of way.)

My mother and I agree: dying is *not* the worst thing that can happen to you. Feeling responsible for someone else's death? That's the most excruciating thing.

And watching someone you dearly love suffer an agonizing death? That's a close second.

And thus, I say again: my own terminal diagnosis barely makes my top five.

What Kind of Child Comes from a Family Like That?

When I was in elementary school, I had a couple of wonderful teachers who kept recommending me to the gifted program, but the principal said, "A gifted child does not come from a family like that." I know this because those teachers were friends with a dear friend of my mother's, also a teacher, who took me out for lunch when I was about twenty-five after I had finished college and taught in Japan for a year or two to tell me the story.

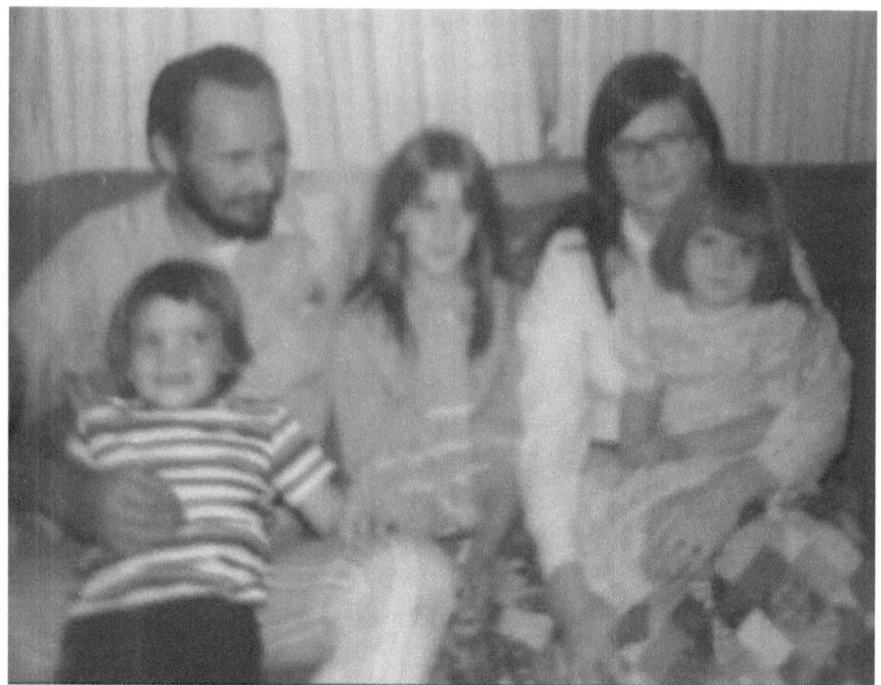

Easter Sunday 1977, Eric George Elisa Dixie Loi

I imagine no one told me before that because they didn't want it to become a self-fulfilling prophecy. Yes, on the basis of my family circumstances, I was denied the advantages that many children from the happier classes enjoyed—at a public school in these United States of America where we boast of equality—liberty and justice for all. We all know some people are more equal than others. Looking back, however, I am so grateful to see that nobody in my family lets other people determine what we are equal to.

My parents treated hardship like an adventure, though, and I will always be grateful for that. They made mistakes, but they did a lot of things right—and one of those was raising us to not be pansies.

To this end, one of their most wonderful gifts was to equip us with the ability to find humor in the worst situations.

In an article I published in the *International Journal of Humor Research* in 2001, I call it *hardship humor* (although my friend Najma called it *hardass humor,* also accurate). It is a sibling to gallows humor.

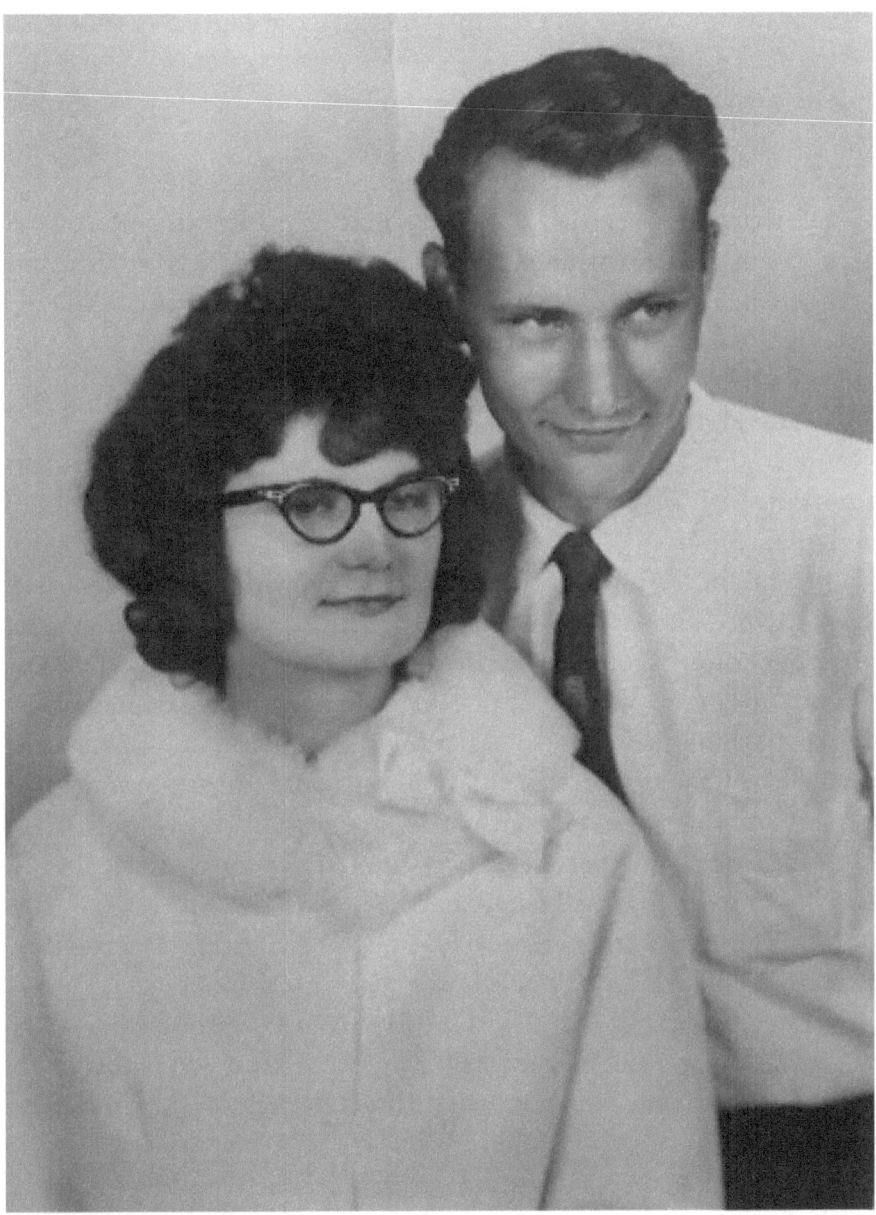

Dixie and George Everts 1965

My blind mother, who raised five children and cooked and cleaned and ironed and gardened and led Girl Scouts and taught children's church and volunteered at nursing homes and was a Mary Kay consultant for ten years, taught me that I can do anything that I have to. Necessity is the mother of bucking up.

So, the first reason I didn't fall apart in the face of cancer? It's not what you know, it's who you know.

I hate to name drop, but Adversity and I grew up together. We are like sisters.

Hello Darkness, my old friend. Suffering is old hat to me.

I feel that I have earned the equivalent of a PhD in suffering. (I think I've already mentioned the not insubstantial credentials of my having spent ten years of my life weeping. And yes, my actual PhD did contribute to that suffering. Thank you for asking).

The Adversity Advantage

John Haidt, in *The Happiness Hypothesis*,[1] writes about the importance of adversity in building emotional and psychological strength.

When I reflected on the equanimity I felt in facing stage IV cancer, it slowly dawned on me: I've kind of evolved into an emotional triathlete.

Not by choice, of course—but I've been training for this my whole life.

I don't mean the purpose of that adversity was to prepare me for *this* adversity. I think the arguments that Matilda-God caused you suffering to prepare you for more of the same or so you could empathize with other people's suffering are more than a little circular.

But the effect of all that adversity was to train and prepare me for this adversity, and I may as well rejoice in that.

In addition to having parents who presented adversity as adventure, my mother joined a Pentecostal church when I was about eight.

Statistically, I think the majority of Pentecostals around the world live on the "wrong side of the tracks," and yet they are the most joyful people I have ever met, and they believe that God has a beautiful plan for everyone.

Thus, I grew up believing that God was absolutely calling me into a wonderful future.

Pentecostals generally believe that anyone can become anything if they collaborate with God in creating their lives. In a way, they are the spiritualized version of the American dream on steroids.[2]

Although self-fulfilling prophecy is not one of their sponsored products, I think the trajectory of my life might be viewed through that lens. In *Atlas of the Heart*,[3] Brené Brown observes that hope is learned.

I learned it from the Pentecostals and am forever grateful. Even though I hurt desperately from a cluster bomb of trauma, I always believed that my wounds would one day be healed, and my needs would be met.

I also believed that I had something to offer the world because God endowed me with something to offer the world (and that this is true for everyone). Since I managed to go on and earn a PhD from Georgetown University even without the early advantage of that prestigious small-town public elementary school gifted program, there may be something to that particular culture of hope.

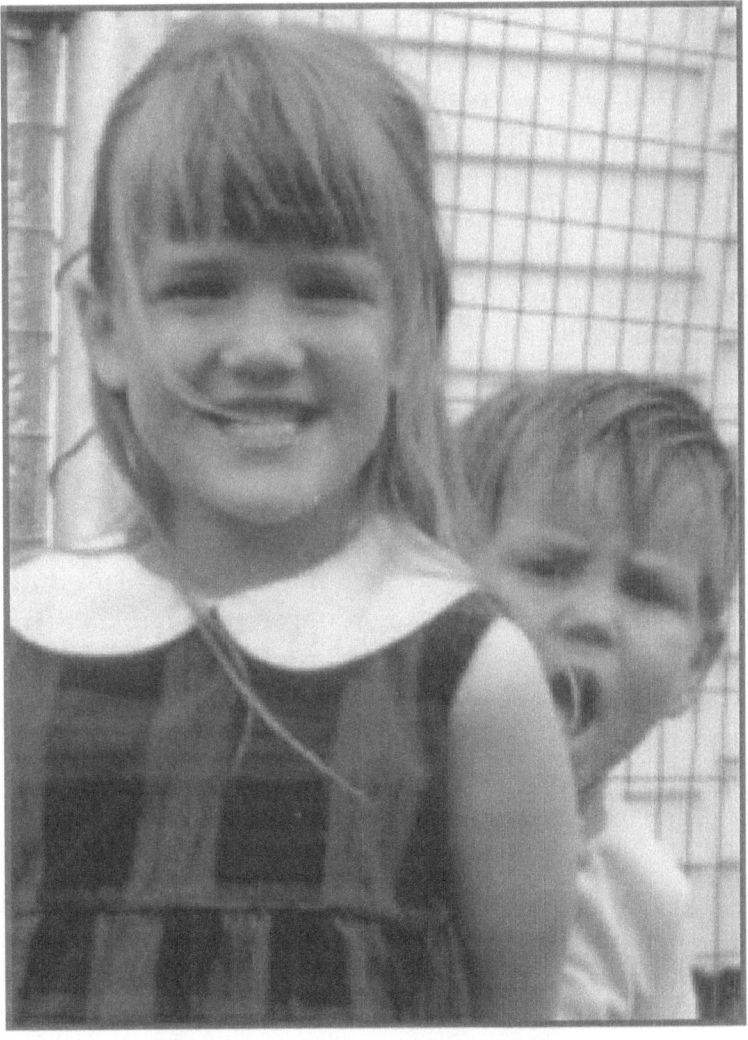

Elisa and Indignant Brian, 1971.

What Are Little Girls Made Of?

Moreover, my father, who considered himself an agnostic and took a very dim view of Pentecostals, nevertheless was also an autodidact and a man of great imagination. (Less charitable family associates would say he lived in a fantasy world, which—duh—is pretty much a defining feature of the manic phase of bipolar disorder.)

Be that as it may, he taught me to dream big dreams. He was always giving me college-level textbooks as a child, and I think this was less because he did not know about stages of child development than because he simply did not feel they applied to his personal offspring.

(They did, by the way. I didn't read most of those books. But they nevertheless contributed to my budding scholarly identity.)

When I was seven, he started teaching me electronics. He had a well-worn study guide for the FCC (Federal Communications Commission) exam that was heavily underlined in red ink and smelled like his cigarettes. This study guide prepared one for a license that would qualify the licensee to operate on the radio, and we studied that together every night.

By day I attended public school, which was generally boring AF, and by night I was privy to the tutelage of my dad, the weirdest supplementary homeschooler ever. I'll note that I didn't have the clearest idea what that license would do for me. Getting to study and take a test were their own reward. (My nerdiness started early.)

When I was eight, I passed that exam and was awarded my third-class FCC license. I'm guessing I was the youngest person to do so in 1975, and I would bet money I was the only little girl.

In fact, the first time I took the exam, I failed, and my father was completely mystified. Not angry, just mystified. It never entered either of our minds that it had anything to do with my being eight.

After I took my exam, I whiled away the time running up the down escalator and experimenting with the novelty of a fascinating vending machine that produced hot soup (it was the '70s), waiting for him to finish his exam (for a first-class license).

I now realize that through this experience, without my even noticing, he taught me that there was no reason that other people's expectations for age, gender, and social class should apply to me.

My mother taught me the same lesson through her own life. Whenever someone told her blind people can't do such-and-such, they really should have been advised to stand back, because they had just thrown gasoline on her fire. She generally took such naysaying as a challenge and proceeded to do whatever it was blind people were allegedly unable to do—if not with the greatest of ease, certainly with a great deal of attitude.

Hide and Watch

My mother wouldn't drink beer if you paid her to, but the spirit of *Hold my beer* could sum up her whole life.

She had her own expression for this (which seems to have originated in the hills of Arkansas, where she spent her early childhood). She loved to say, especially to us children, "Hide and watch." Not sure why the hiding was necessary, but it does make it funnier, so it worked on several levels. I have come to believe that it was our unofficial family motto. If you tell us we can't do something, we will take that as a challenge and respond in attitude with, "Hide and watch."

So, like I said, I don't want to brag, but when it comes to facing adversity like cancer, through no real agency of my own, I went to the best possible prep school. And when my first oncologist told me I had a 5% chance of having fun in the year ahead, I invoked the family motto and inwardly replied, *Hide and watch.*

And in my blind mother's Arkansas bravado, I thought, *Well, now we'll find out what this little girl is made of.* And largely thanks to my eccentric and exceptional parents, I lucked out with better fare than sugar and spice and everything nice.

And that's a darned good thing, because if I'd been made of weaker mettle, the real adversity ahead of me—not cancer, but complicated grief—would have completely destroyed me instead of just almost destroying me.

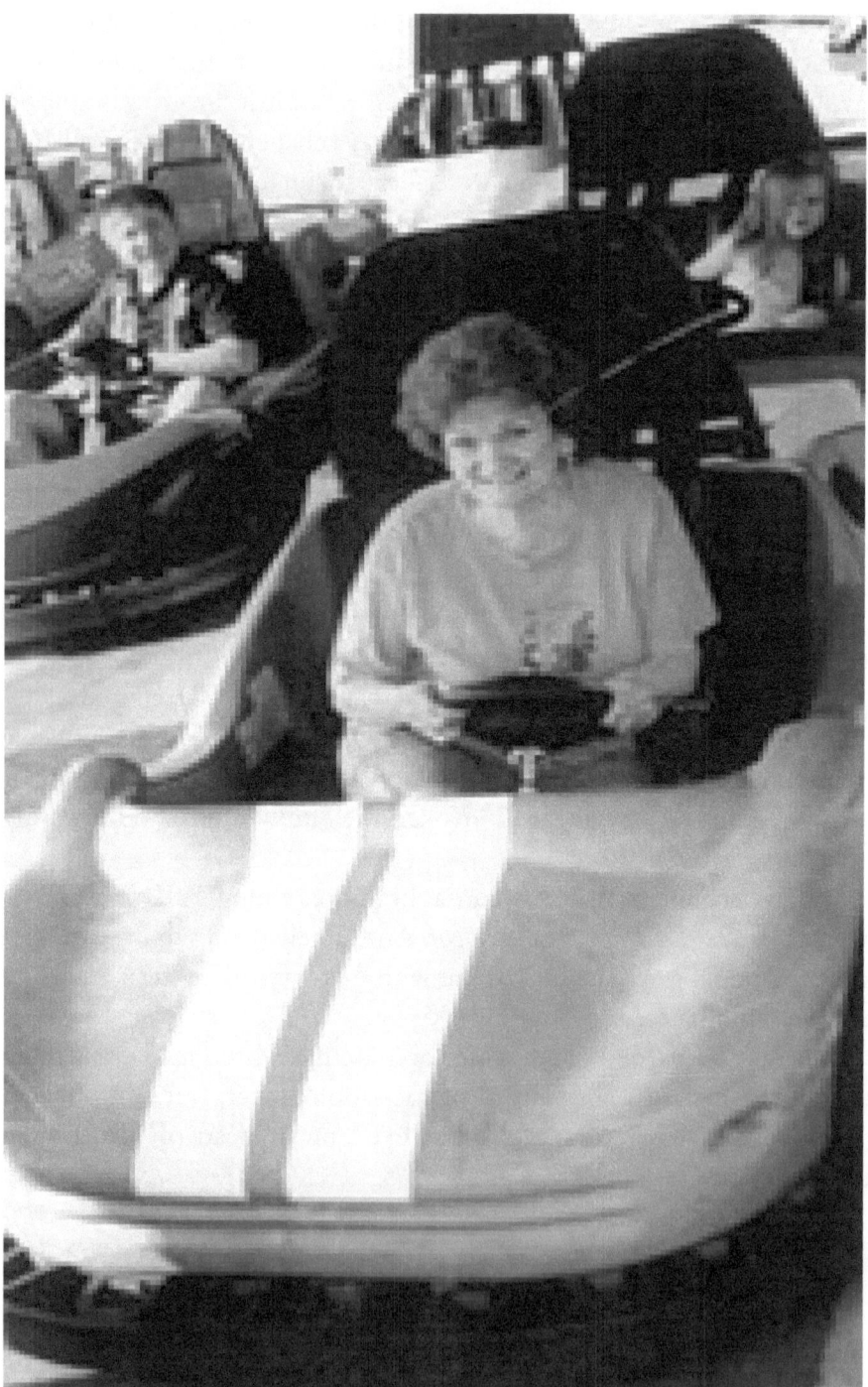

Mom in a Bumper Car with the Grands around 2002, completely blind by this time.

1. Haidt, Jonathan. *The Happiness Hypothesis: Finding Modern Truth in Ancient Wisdom*. Basic Books, 2006.

2. In my experience, Pentecostals differ from prosperity gospel adherents in that classic Pentecostals embrace suffering along with blessing.

3. Brown, Brené. *Atlas of the Heart: Mapping Meaningful Connection and the Language of Human Experience*. Random House, 2021.

6

How Could Anyone Grieve for 50 years?

Well, I'm so glad you asked. Now, having explained where much of my resilience came from, I want to explain how I nevertheless got broken to smithereens before getting healed.

"Hide and watch" is an energy I wish I had pulsing through me throughout my life. Some experiences are so soul-crushing, however, that no amount of bravado can simply power you through.

There is grief that is like a simple fracture, and then there are compound fractures of the soul—like mine—where your bone is broken in multiple places and sticking out of your flesh. That metaphor, like the story I'm about to tell you, is hard to read. I'm sorry. It was even harder to live.

I believe some of you have also experienced compound fractures of the soul, and it is for you, most of all, that I write my story.

There are several kinds of grief that can be especially hard to rise out of. Some of these include *disenfranchised grief, complicated grief, traumatic grief,* and *early childhood grief*—each of which is a tremendous challenge, and all of which hit me right between the eyes simultaneously.

Disenfranchised Grief
Disenfranchised Grief is the experience of loss that isn't openly acknowledged, socially supported, or publicly mourned. When the relationship, the loss, or even the griever isn't seen as valid, the pain often goes unrecognized, leaving the mourner feeling isolated and silenced.

I experienced this when my brother died. In cases of a child's death, people tend to focus solely on the parents' grief. Surviving siblings become an afterthought.

Later, when my dear friend Diane died, I encountered it again. She wasn't biological family, just "a friend," and no one around me seemed to understand the depth of my grief (except my mother). No one knew Diane, and no one cared.

I was in graduate school then, surrounded by people who, understandably, didn't feel responsible for my sorrow. Still, in both cases, I was utterly alone in my bereavement.

Complicated Grief

Complicated Grief, also known as *Prolonged Grief Disorder*, isn't just grief that lingers—it's grief that digs in, sends its roots deep into your soul, and won't let go. It's the kind of mourning where the pain doesn't ease over time, where the loss doesn't fade—if anything, it calcifies.

It can make daily life feel unmanageable, because you're not just grieving the person—you're also struggling to adjust to many emotional, psychological, spiritual, and even physical complications.

Because I was there—present and involved—when my brother died, I experienced one of the most intense and tangled versions of complicated grief. It wasn't just sadness. It was the agony of loss woven together with shame, guilt, self-blame—emotions that settle into the body instead of moving through it, that can distort your sense of self and make healing feel out of reach.

Traumatic Grief

There's also *Traumatic Grief*—the kind that comes from sudden, violent loss, like a child being hit by a truck. That kind of shock doesn't just hurt; it shatters. You're left picking up fragments of memory, mind, and identity, trying to process horror, helplessness, and senselessness.

For me, it came with a brutally direct form of survivor's guilt—unrelenting, and impossible to identify or articulate as a child. Honestly, it was more than survivor's guilt. I believed that I was actually responsible for his death.

Psychologically, this kind of grief can bring flashbacks, intrusive images, hypervigilance, and that never-ending sense that the other shoe is about to drop. You might feel numb or on edge, emotionally detached, unable to sleep, plagued by nightmares, unable to concentrate or make decisions. You're flooded with guilt and fear.

The year before I started trauma therapy, I went to get tested for ADHD. At the time, I was teaching at Texas A&M, and some of my students thought I might have ADHD because of the nonlinear nature of some of my speech and thought patterns. After two hours of evaluation, the psychologist looked at me and said, "You don't have ADHD. You have trauma. And there's no medicine for that."

That fragmentation—the shattering—affects not just the mind but the nervous system. Your body carries it too. I've lived with fibromyalgia since childhood, which worsened in adulthood. I ended up in the ER with stomach pain several times—once with acute appendicitis, but other times they just told me it was IBS. Exhaustion, headaches, breathlessness—grief plays havoc on the nervous system.

Emotionally, traumatic grief isn't just sadness. It's prolonged despair. Rage. Isolation. Sometimes, you avoid anything that reminds you of them because the reminders cut too deep. Sometimes you spiral into depression, anxiety, or full-blown PTSD.

There are risks—of self-harm, of suicidal thoughts, of choosing numbness wherever you can find it. In my late twenties, I drank heavily to quiet the pain. Later, I combined alcohol with medication—an accidental overdose would've been so easy.

And then there's what happens to your beliefs, your sense of meaning, your trust in the world. Grief like this shakes the foundation of who you are. It makes you question everything you thought was solid: your purpose, your faith, your safety, your identity.

While some people turn away from God, I turned into God. Some might have called my faith at that time pure fanaticism. Maybe it was. And maybe it saved me.

Early Childhood Grief

When grief begins in early childhood, it becomes something else entirely—more complicated, more hidden. Children don't yet have the tools to grieve. They can't name their pain, so their grief shows up in behavior: in acting out, in withdrawal, in fear.

I was one of those children. I didn't understand what had happened, but my amygdala—the brain's fear center—did.

Early trauma like that rewires the brain. It leaves deep emotional imprints: hypervigilance, chronic anxiety, and later, depression, PTSD, even attachment disorders.

I didn't just carry my brother's death. I carried its aftermath in my nervous system for decades.

I had nightmares. I couldn't sleep through the night. My teachers would write on my report cards, "Elisa has the potential to get straight A's, but she does not apply herself."

I couldn't think. If only they knew everything I was applying myself to.

The Whole Enchilada

I was hit by the full brunt of all four of these types of grief with Brian's death—and both traumatic and complicated grief with Diane's death.

I suffered from most of the effects I've listed. I think it was analogous to having compound fractures in multiple limbs. And I would argue that such wounds to the soul are even harder to heal than such wounds to the body.

Though, as I write in one poem about the experience, with truly deft cruelty, not one mark is left on the body; these wounds are completely invisible.

As a child (and as an adult), my wounds were unseen, and I was unable to advocate for myself. Having cemented this experience into my psyche, I continued unable to advocate for myself for many, many years.

Not to fear. I eventually found a psychiatrist who saw exactly what the problem was and took me through a process of trauma therapy that healed the mother wound.

It took several more years for the healing to complete itself, but it did.

I used to want to die regularly and suffered constantly from depression. Today, I am so happy and so whole. I never want to die. I don't suffer from depression, and I delight in my life and the lovely people in it.

I write this story from the other side of healing. I want you to know that, in my experience, even deep, long-lasting trauma can be healed.

— • —

PART II: THE FIRST TIME CANCER TRIED TO WRECK MY LIFE (SHE SUCCEEDED)

7

— • —

DYING TOGETHER

Point of Reference

Have you already had encounters with cancer or death? If you have, that experience has no doubt deeply colored your view and your expectations. It kind of creates a script you unwittingly follow.

That was true for me, too. The first time cancer tried to wreck my life—when my friend Diane died—it absolutely succeeded. And that experience was my point of reference, my knowledge base.

I have been largely jocular and lighthearted up till this point, but now I am going to take a sharp turn and take you into my darkest night so you can see the cancer that shaped me, that chewed me up and spit me out but ultimately led to the healing that enables me to be jocular and lighthearted.

I need to tell you about the agony that has mauled and molded my soul.

The poet and spiritual luminary Rumi, as I mentioned in Chapter One, writes that you have to die before you die,[1] which I think is not too different from the Christian idea of dying to self and which is a necessary precondition to personal resurrection.

I think it also might be related to the Buddhist idea of nonattachment. Once you release certain attachments you are free.

My experience with Diane is how I died before I died. I suppose it helped me to be less attached to both life and death when I was given a terminal diagnosis.

The blog post I'm about to share was my attempt to explain to my beloveds why I did not want to pursue treatment for stage IV pancreatic cancer. In it, I return to Diane's death—an experience that gutted me in my early thirties.

You might wonder why I don't begin with my childhood loss and move forward chronologically. That's a fair question.

The truth is, I didn't realize my childhood loss had left such a deep wound until I began unraveling the complicated grief I carried after Diane died.

So, I'm telling the story not in the order in which events happened, but in the order in which they revealed themselves to me.

Let Me Explain My Attitude Towards Pancreatic Cancer
June 6, 2020

I know that some of you are disappointed, maybe even appalled, by my response to learning I have metastatic pancreatic cancer (and refusing treatment). You feel that I have given up before the fight has even begun. I have not "given up," Loves. I will fight for a quality of life as long as I can, and I will live it with gusto! But I am a realist. I can't help thinking of Westley saying in *The Princess Bride*, "We are men of action. Lies do not become us."[2] Let me help you understand my heart and how it got this way.

It was my beloved Diane whose gruesome death by stomach cancer in 2001 shaped my experience and understanding of hard cancers. I will share this view with you, first by way of letters I have written to her long after her death, so that you may understand why I think the way I do.

Retrospective Letter #1

My Dear Diane, You were the most beautiful chapter of my college years (and that's saying something, because those were beautiful years). I am at a loss when I try to describe our friendship to others. You were like a missing piece of my soul, and when I met you, it clicked right into place.

I was like your older sister, helping you adjust to life in the United States in general (your having grown up in Belgium) and at our little Pentecostal college in particular. And you adored me as much as I adored you. I felt like no one had ever loved me so much in my life. I remember you exclaiming one day, "Where have you been all my life?!" You were the source of such exquisite joy.

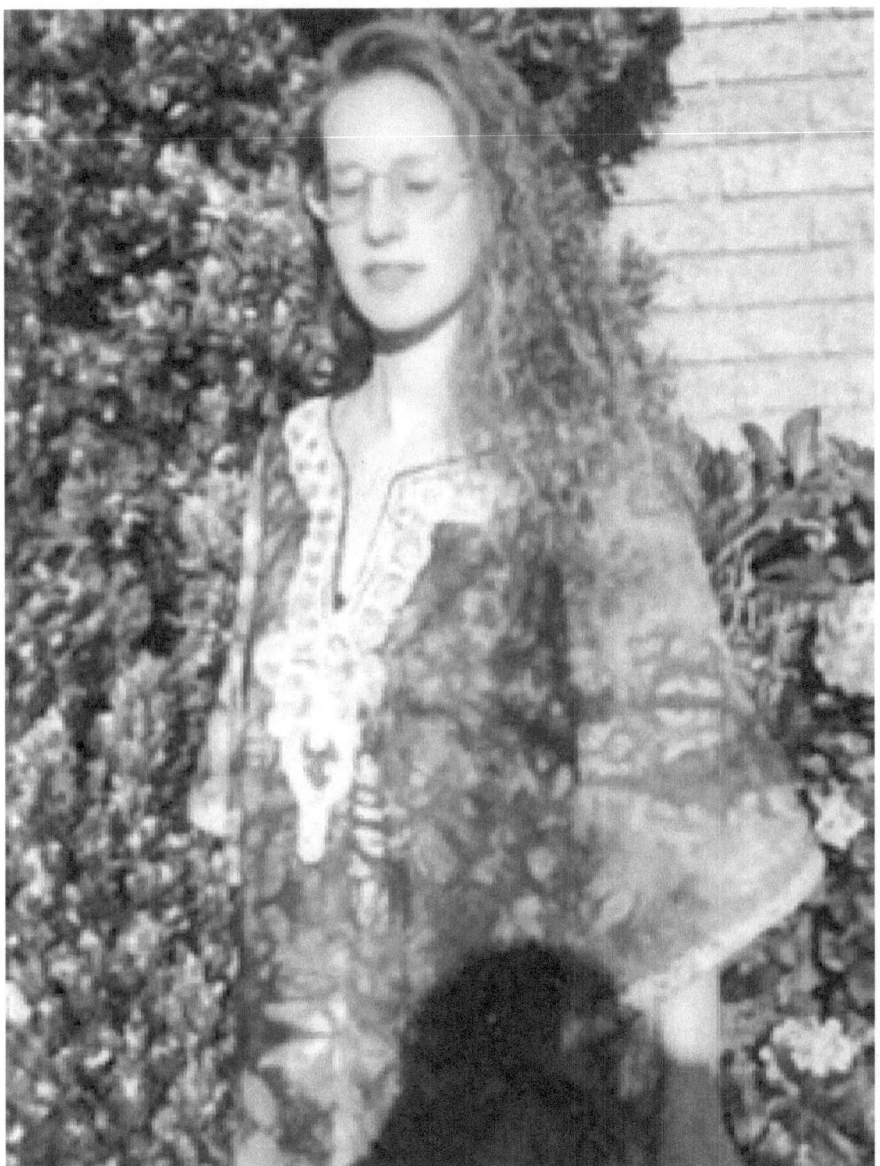

Diane in South Africa eyes closed with Hydrangeas dying in the background, a foreshadowing

No one told me that two people who had been so very close could, in just five years [from 1990–1995], grow so far apart that the people they used to be virtually disappeared—and their intimate connection with them. I would not have believed or understood it had I not lived it.

I suppose, however, that it is also because we were so young, and had yet to understand the way life would wear us into different shapes as the years passed—in some ways lovely, in others grotesque, like driftwood battered against the waves. No two pieces ever worn in the same way.

But what else did we anticipate? It wasn't just five years apart after a painful separation; it was five years apart on different sides of the planet, in foreign cultures which could hardly have been more disparate—Japan and South Africa.

Perhaps I should rather wonder at the deep connection that remained, however difficult to describe. Perhaps it was at some barely fathomable spiritual level that we were still one soul with two hearts.

When I gazed into your eyes, I still found myself at home there, and I trust you felt the same—even though we had changed all the furniture and nearly all the art on the walls of our souls.

There was so much to learn from each other that we never learned. We didn't know enough to see this. We didn't know enough to ask.

I only learned in your final weeks that a four-year-old child had died in your arms on the way to the hospital in South Africa! How had we never talked about that??

I was so alarmed to learn this—and so alarmed that I had not already known. I was so alarmed at how little I still knew of you after twelve years.

Your Love for South Africa

I don't know that I ever told you how much I always admired—and marveled at—how deeply you had loved South Africa since you were three years old and first learned about apartheid while living in Belgium.

From that incredibly tender age, you wanted to act, to do something in solidarity, alongside black South Africans. That desire burned in your heart all your life.

So, I was delighted—and not at all surprised—when your family got the opportunity to leave Belgium as a mission field and move to South Africa, where your father would serve as dean of another Bible school. Influenced by your great love, they did.

And as you had just completed your B.A. at our illustrious Pentecostal "liberal" arts college, you went to join them. I was still in Japan and learned of these developments through your precious letters.

I was so proud of you for working at a shelter for homeless, orphaned young girls in Cape Town for four years. I love to tell people about how every morning on your way to work you passed and greeted Desmond Tutu having tea.

You threw your maternal compassion and tenderness into that noble endeavor—into loving those dear girls with the purest of hearts.

Until one day, the news came that your own blind mother's cancer had returned.

And you were obliged to join your family in Johannesburg to care for her for a year as she lay dying.

Your Own Point of Reference

The palliative care was horrendous, and the death she died—horrific. She had seizures that were almost as traumatic for you as they were for her.

In spite of the agony, she died as quietly as she could, with the grace of a martyr. She was buried in Johannesburg, in a pine coffin, in solidarity with the poor and disenfranchised of South Africa—especially those dying of AIDS.

And you returned to the States with your lonely, little grief-wearied, broken-hearted family—your father and your little brother—for a year, to raise funds to return to the mission field.

While you were still in South Africa, my four years in Japan had come to a precipitous end, and I moved to Chicago (since after one has lived in the largest city in the world, she can never really go back to Kansas).

Marvelously, your family came back for your year of furlough to be based in Chicago, too. Remember when I met you all at the airport and drove you to the missionary housing waiting for you?

I was deeply pleased to see you, though I was shocked by the Diane who returned to me. Five brief years had changed you so dramatically.

What did the gruesome death of your mother do to your faith, my love? What did it do to your heart and to your soul?

It seemed to have torn you into pieces and to have left you with thick, hard scars.

It changed you in horrible ways. Grief sometimes makes people more tender, but it made you brittle beyond belief—beyond what I would have imagined possible from such a tender, joyful soul.

You had been so effervescent, so full of life and *joie de vivre!* These were your hallmarks.

Now you seemed but a shell of your former self. You were still beautiful, but so broken and subdued—and sharp-edged.

Ending Up In the Same Town

I was pleased that you decided to stay in Chicago and pursue a Master's in Missions at Trinity. I was doing a Master's in Linguistics at Northeastern.

Remember how we would meet up periodically, almost as casual friends would do? I tried some of the churches you went to, attended with you some weeks, had lunch after.

You especially liked to meet on Mother's Day and your mother's birthday because I was the only person in Chicago (after your family went back to South Africa) who had known your mother.

We would have lunch and then take long walks, talking about her, and then about all the happenings of our lives.

Although dancing had been forbidden for us growing up Pentecostal, you were becoming more ecumenical, and your code had changed.

You shared with me the amazing phenomenon of your becoming a swing dancer—and not just any swing dancer, but a really good one!

Since we were raised to believe that dancing was sinful, this was truly remarkable, and I rejoiced with you.

After these talks, we would hug, say, "I love you," and go our separate ways. Almost perfunctorily.

Oh, my beloved, what happened to us?

The Devastating News

I got my fellowship to do my doctorate and moved to DC. Email was new! My first ever account was at Northeastern, and I had neglected to check it the whole time I was away my first semester, so it was the first thing I checked when I got to Chicago.

I was stunned to find an email from your father. There was no beating around the bush. He had written to inform me that you had stomach cancer, but this email had been sitting in my inbox for months.

An icy shiver of doom and terror swept through my body, leaving my bones cold and my own stomach aching. Of the handful of people I knew of who had had stomach cancer, all of them had died swiftly, within a few months of diagnosis. Not one had survived.

I knew that you would not survive either. Always the pragmatist (no, I cannot yet explain how I can be equally pragmatist and idealist—for an analog of this mystery I direct you to the doctrine of the Trinity), I braced myself for the end.

If you're going to die, you must prepare. There is a lot of work to do before you can leave your life the way you want to.

I thought of myself as being a realist. Others thought of my approach, I think, as being an emissary (if not a cheerleader) for the Grim Reaper. I'm afraid you were one of these, my dear.

I do not believe in pretending. I have always been the cut-through-the-crap friend who tells you the truth when asked. You knew that all too well.

I have to admit, however, that I was afraid of seeing you for the first time after this earth-shattering news. I marshaled our mutual friend Brian to go with me to visit you.

Although your church group was praying for your healing, even as a Pentecostal at that time, I was not one to put much stock in faith healers. I believe miracles are exceedingly rare (something about having a blind mother who was prayed over hundreds of times over the course of decades without any change).

So, I knew in my bones you were going to die, and soon. I don't know what I said during that visit, but I said something that betrayed this belief.

Brian tried to cover for me, but all I could think about was what you would be facing and all you would need to do before you died. I have never been good at denial (well, except for one tiny, enormous detail, but I will leave that for another time).

And after that first "slip," you would not look into my eyes. You would look at me more diffusely, without focus. I sought your gaze, but if our eyes met for a fraction of a second, yours would dart away.

Knowing that stomach cancer is swift, and you and your family seemed to be either in complete denial or complete ignorance about that, I made the twelve-hour trip to Chicago five times that year, thinking each time might be the last time that I saw you, my sweet girl, this side of Jordan.

Unfortunately for you, my love, I do not have the gift of being able to lie with my eyes. You knew what I thought and what I saw, and you studiously avoided looking me in the eye every time we met.

I wanted you to prepare for the end. You wanted to deny that there would ever be an end.

I missed our honest gaze so much, I even had dreams in which the most arresting feature was just you actually looking me in the eye and communing with me in that intimate way we used to have.

I am so sorry that I could not manufacture hope for you. It seemed like you had a lot of other people trying to do that.

I think my gift was being able to navigate in the dark. What I wanted was to be able to walk through the Valley of the Shadow of Death with you, and no one who was still in denial would ever be able to do that.

I shall love you always.

Reflection

Almost twenty-five years later, I still wonder—can you die with someone if you don't actually physically expire yourself?

But I did not want her walking that path alone.

And I was determined to walk down that road with her as far as I possibly could.

Right up to death's door.

---

1. Rumi. *The Masnavi*, Book VI, lines 754-758. Translated by Camille Adams Helminski and Kabir Helminski, *Rumi: Daylight*, Shambhala, 1999.

2. *The Princess Bride*. Directed by Rob Reiner, screenplay by William Goldman, performance by Cary Elwes, 20th Century Fox, 1987.

8

— ⋅ —

CHERRY BLOSSOMS

I t's amazing how easy it is to plow through our days unthinkingly, barely noticing that we are alive.

I wonder what experiences in your life have made you stop and see how precious your life is. Did Death have to punch you in the face, or were there subtler invitations that awakened your awareness?

I'll never know whether I might have been sensitive to the gentler approach, since Death chose the violent one with me.

However I got ushered into this holy place though, I am grateful. Not that my loved ones died, but that I got to be near them.

The shadow of death is a sacred, holy place. It is a thin space where you feel very near the divine.

Cherish These Blossoms While You May

June 6, 2020

One of the gifts of cancer is that it shines a magnifying glass on your life and your connections to the people who matter most to you.

You suddenly attend to details you hadn't been noticing. You sort through your experiences; you examine your patterns, appraise your relationships.

I learned so much about how I wanted to live by watching my young friend, Diane, die. I studied her life and her death and let them inform my own.

One thing I learned was how to cherish the moment we are in right now—the present—so much of which will be swept away by the wind tomorrow.

Retrospective Letter #2

My Dear Diane, I don't know how much experience you have of viewing cherry blossoms, Love; I never thought to ask. Living in Japan for four years, I got to see a lot of them and to celebrate them with my Japanese friends season after season. A grove of cherry blossom trees all in bloom is a breathtaking affair, but perhaps the most beautiful element is the carpet of delicate petals that covers the ground beneath the canopy of pink and white above.

That carpet can only be made as the blossoms begin to die.

You walk into such a grove like walking into some kind of floral, arboreal womb, wrapped up in the cycle of life, all this safety and warmth and oneness with Mother Earth. Above your head, life shouting and singing such glory, and beneath your feet, the sweet quiet rest of the flowers' demise. Is it more like a womb or a tomb? I can see it both ways.

The carpet of petals looks like a kind of snow. And there is a hushed tone in this space, the way the first day of blanketing snow hushes a city and its neighborhoods. Whether womb or tomb, a miraculous quiet. A sacred place of awe. The Japanese are right to celebrate this glory so religiously.

Oh, my dearest, how differently we remember the spring of 2001, I am almost ashamed. You experiencing chemo, trying to keep your food down and your hope up. My heart was dichotomized. Sometimes I sobbed for you uncontrollably (this even happened to me in public once at Georgetown and it was quite a scene!). But somehow, I was often able to keep my sorrow for you in one place, and my academic progress somewhere else entirely.

I was in so many ways at the top of my game, in many ways, at the top of my life! I was doing so well in graduate school at Georgetown in a department which is number one in the world, bar none, for what we do. It was an experience I considered an outrageous gift of grace.

I'm not sure if I told you about these circumstances (which I realize are utterly mundane compared to what was happening to you). I had just organized a double session panel for an important conference in my field. It was a wonderful opportunity, and I was thrilled to be doing it, but of course it was attended by an equal proportion of stress and responsibility.

I had to amalgamate all the elaborate applications of ten people, who, unsurprisingly, being human, all submitted at the last possible minute, about 2:00 p.m. on the day everything was due. And I then had to physically take this pile of materials to the conference headquarters that, for this year, was across the bridge in Arlington, Virginia. All due on this day in April at 4:00 p.m.

I managed to get it all done and rushed to my car parked on 34th Street (near Madeleine Albright's house), and there it was—with a boot on it. I had never had a boot before, had not the faintest idea what to do about a boot.

So, I trudged back to campus in desperation and fortuitously ran into my friend Karen, who had a car and time to take me to the conference headquarters in Arlington, and then to the DMV downtown (which was a pretty scary affair at that time—in a part of the city where I didn't feel very safe).

Anyway, a few hours and $150.00 later, after all these hurdles were cleared, Karen drove me back to my car to wait for the mythical boot people, who said they would come and unboot it within two hours, and so I sent her home.

Reflections Under the Cherry Blossom Tree

I walked over to campus to sit beneath a glorious cherry blossom tree in full bloom and meditate while I waited. I was so relieved to have all the conference application process done. I could sit and soak up the beauty of spring—the beauty of these evanescent blossoms, with their delicate petals that would come and go in a flash, but would return faithfully every spring, year after year.

In the spring of 2000, just the year before, I had had a crushing experience with that little group of friends I was introduced to through you. They were a little embryonic church plant. I had let myself be grafted into that group like a grafted branch grows into a tree. I loved them and cherished the hopeful vision they shared. But in the end, it became toxic through a spectacular failure of egocentric leadership, and I had to amputate myself from it.

Eventually, everyone did. The little family we had created among us disbanded and died. One of the (good) pastors called it *group euthanasia*. I had invested so much in those relationships and in our dreams for the future, and I cried for so many months.

That year, I had sat under this very same tree, wondering in dismay at how everything that blossoms also dies.

But I had lived.

And now, here I was again—so close to whole. I rested and reveled in the fact that the seasons come 'round year after year. Seasons of barrenness and crushing pain, of bitterness and *bewilderness*, followed by seasons of healing and renewal, of rebirth and joy and laughter.

Faithfully, season after season.

And I was content.

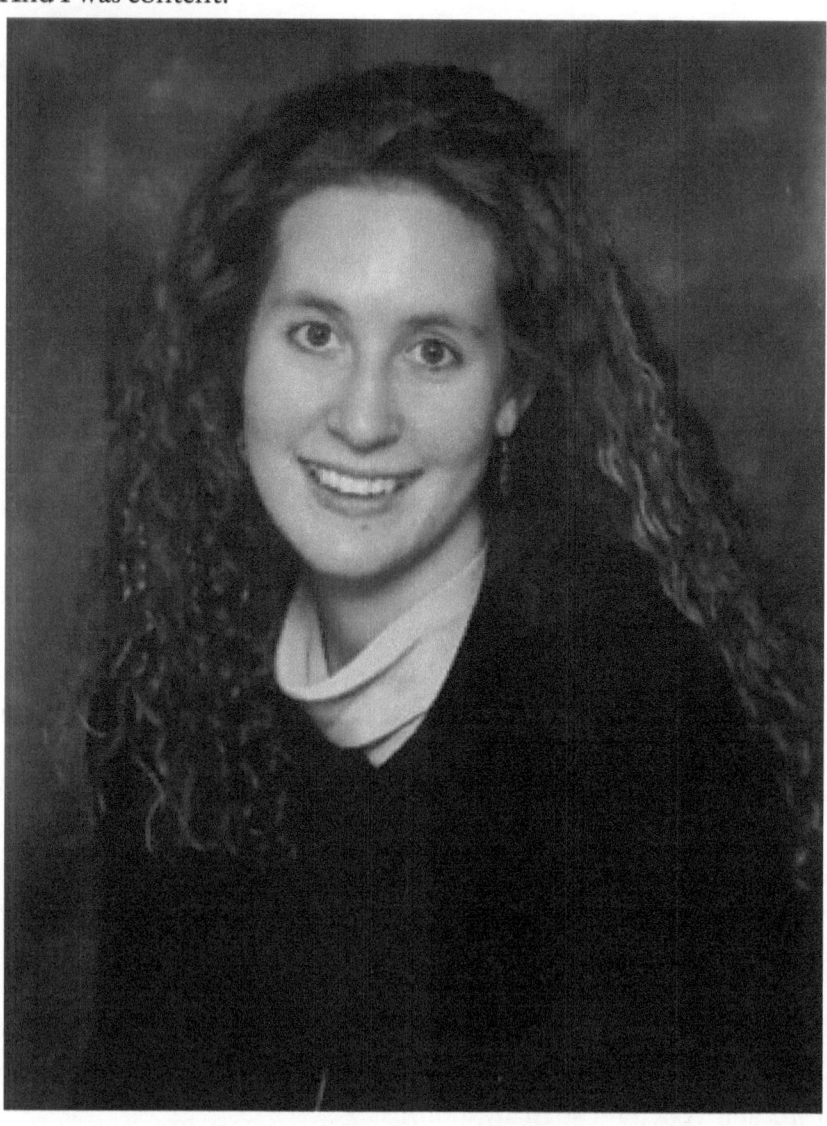

I believe this was taken the year before Diane died.

Crossing the Bridge

After that worshipful little moment under the cherry blossom tree, I strolled back to my car. And there it was—unfettered, unshackled, free as the seagulls soaring over earth and bay. My tangible little metaphor.

I drove home across the Potomac, past the Georgetown crew rowing vigorously upriver, past the bright new sprigs of green lifting their thousands of little arms in worship against the gray sky. And all was well with the world. All glorious. All victorious.

I parked, rode the elevator to my fifteenth-floor apartment, walked into the kitchen, and pressed play on the answering machine.

It was your voice, my sweet girl.

You said, "The cancer is back. They don't think I have long."

I dropped everything I was carrying and sank to my knees.

I could already see my cherry blossom begin her descent.

Your lovely petals would soon fall gracefully to the ground until you disappeared. Sure, there would be other blossoms in the years and seasons to come. But never again would there be this blossom. You had to be cherished in the moment and to know that you were cherished.

My dearest Diane Cheri, it grieved me so much to learn that you did not know how much I have always cherished you, until I came to die with you.

I Didn't Know You Loved Me This Much

June 14, 2020

When Diane began her—let's say—*ascent*, and I was making preparations to go care for her, a mutual acquaintance expressed surprise:

"The last I heard, you weren't very happy with Diane."

I was taken aback. Like—what does that have to do with the price of (adorably hedgehog-decorated COVID) masks in China?? How does not being happy with someone have *anything* to do with how much you love them?

It was Easter 2001 when I made my fifth trip from D.C. to Chicago, thinking it might be the last time I saw her. She told me the cancer was "back" (she was in denial—it had never left), and she was preparing for another surgery.

Her father and stepmother were there, but when the weekend ended, they simply returned to their library jobs in Minnesota, leaving her in

ICU—alone. She had nightmares of dead bodies and meat hanging in freezers (and the poor girl was a vegetarian).

I couldn't leave her like that.

So, I extended my Easter break by a week and asked my friends at Georgetown if they could give my final presentations for me. They kindly agreed. And my professors—bless them—weren't annoyed at all. They were proud of me. That's one of the reasons I love that department so much.

One of our most precious moments came after a minor procedure. I walked into her hospital room and reached out to take her hand. As she extended hers, she noticed with dismay that there was blood on it and began to pull away.

I laughed and said, *"It doesn't matter, honey,"* and took that soft, beloved hand into my own.

She promptly fell asleep.

And I stood there, leaning over her bed, awkwardly holding that hand for a very long time—not wanting to disturb her rest, and honestly, not wanting to lose that connection. Ever.

When I told her about it later, she said, *"That is so sweet."* And I said, *"Well, it was collaboratively constructed sweetness,"*—in the geek speak of my discipline. She was highly amused.

Pearls of Great Price

In a day or so, Diane was able to sit up in a chair. I was organizing her gifts and flowers on the other side of the room, and she was quiet for a bit. I asked her what she was thinking about, and she looked up and said, "The value of true friends." And I smiled and said, *"I know. A true friend is like a pearl of great price..."* She continued the verse, *"And when you find that pearl..."* And together we finished, *"...you sell everything you have to get that pearl."*

At the end of that visit, I left her a small gift on which I simply addressed her as *Pearl.*

Later, she would say to me in wonder and disbelief, "I didn't know you loved me this much."

Oh my God, what heartbreaking words. After twelve years of friendship—of connection, separation, silence, and reunion—I had failed to convey the depth of my love. To be fair, there were complications. And maybe there had never been the right moment to show her. But still, my soul was shaken by those words.

"I didn't know you loved me this much."

Oh, my Beloveds—may these words never be true of anyone you love.

If there is someone for whom you would lay everything aside to walk with them on their final journey, tell them.

If there is someone for whom you would take a bullet or give your kidney, do not go the length of your life without expressing to them the depth of your love.

You do not know the number of anyone's days—not yours, not theirs.

How tragic would it be for someone you adore to die never having received this knowledge, this sacred truth: that they were wholly, fiercely, and forever loved.

Write them a letter. Take them for a walk. Zoom them. Sing to them. Tell them.

Whatever you do, make sure they never have reason to say, "I didn't know you loved me this much." Or worse—never get the chance to say it at all because they never learned it.

Do Not Let Heaven Slip Away

My dear ones, I feel like God strategically picks the people She wants us to love, lovingly places them in our paths to discover with delight. It's not like something you choose intellectually. Your heart pulls towards certain people, and you have no real agency in that. Or perhaps that is only the way it works with some of us, I don't know. Or just me. You do have agency in how you respond to those people.

And sometimes I think God peoples my world with so many souls to love, my head spins. The wondering child in the candy store. Heaven is here. And each a heaven unto herself, the main way I think God lavishes upon us. And heaven help us if we let these extravagant gifts slip through our fingers while we are focused on other things.

When I was five and swimming in the Hudson River in upstate New York, when it was swimmable in the early seventies, my beach ball slipped back into the water when I was putting my clothes back on. My mother was telling me to go grab it and I could not quite process that I needed to stop putting my clothes on and go get the ball before it floated away forever.

And of course, that's what happened. It drifted so far out to the horizon... but I thought, *My dad can swim for miles! Why can't he just cruise out there and retrieve it?* But no. He could not retrieve it now. They said some little girl in China would be enjoying it soon, and I was partly mollified at the thought.

What if the people in your life are your heaven and you are so busy putting your pants on that you miss them entirely? The good is the enemy of the best. We can crowd our lives with so many good things that we deprive ourselves of the best things.

What a tragedy if we crowded the heaven out of our lives because we couldn't process that we needed to stop doing what we're doing if we don't want it to slip away like water running down a drain we failed to plug. Or like a beach ball drifting out to sea.

9

FALLING INTO A GREAT WOUND

If you have never watched someone you love suffer on a grand scale, I hope you never do. It is generally far worse than suffering yourself.

That would be why terrorists have more success getting information from a subject by torturing their companion than the subject themselves.

For some of us, it becomes really hard to separate the suffering of the other from one's own.

I am one of these.

Firehose of Grief

While Diane was dying, I was a firehose of grief. I gushed agony. I woke up crying, cried myself to sleep, had nightmares about her, woke crying again.

The first time I went to see her in the hospital at Easter of 2001, they told me that she was hooked up to the breathing tube and the nasal gastric tube and that if she cried it could be life threatening, so I should not cry in front of her.

I was pretty sure I could not pull that off, so I gave them a CD of some Portuguese choral singing (*Madredeus*) to give her and went home. She was disappointed when she learned I was there but didn't come in to see her.

The next day, I did better.

After that I came every day, but I cried hard and would have to run out of the room and cry in the hallway, just racking sobs. Of course, this was distressing to her, but I had no control over it.

I finally got to the point where I would cry until I got to the hospital and the moment I went through the doors I stopped crying and did not cry in front of her all day, eight to twelve hours, and then as soon as I went out of the hospital doors at night I would start crying again until I fell asleep.

When I walked, I literally, physically staggered under the weight of the grief, like a drunk person.

The People Around Her Did Not Get It

Fortuitously, one of my best friends, Judy, lived five minutes away from the hospital Diane was in, so I was blessed to be able to stay with her and her family throughout this ordeal. They are orthodox Jews and Larry told me I was doing a *mitzvah*. A good deed.

I had never been so disappointed in Christians, however. Diane's church was a pretty large one, but mostly full of young people without children. Very few mothers. I think the mothers in a church drive its caregiving because they understand what is involved in keeping another human alive and healthy.

Apparently, there had been round-the-clock care for her when she was going through chemo, but it seemed to me that when it became apparent that Diane was going to die, people scurried back into the light and largely left her.

People who have never needed care or been close to someone who has apparently do not realize that just because you are in the hospital does not mean a nurse is standing by your bed waiting to intervene every time you vomit all over your nasal gastro tubes and face and body and gown and bed.

And when you have stomach cancer, that can happen many, many times a day. And it can be life threatening. Someone needs to be there. And no one was. Not the boyfriend, not the father, not the stepmother, and not one damned person from that church.

At Easter her family had left her in ICU and gone back to another state. She felt totally abandoned. That's why I extended my break and stayed through the next weekend.

I had absolutely no use for that boyfriend. He rarely visited her and did not participate in caregiving. That's not love. On the few occasions when he did stay with her for a few hours, she told me he just pushed the button and called for the nurse every time there was a need.

She was quite capable of pushing the button herself. He promised to take her to the lake, for a picnic, various things which he never did. She waited for him for hours and hours every day and most days, he never even showed up.

I wanted to wring his neck.

The last day before I was to come back to DC, I stayed with her all day, went home to take a nap, and then came back to spend the night with her and then leave for my twelve-hour trip home in the morning.

When I came in, I had to come through a different door and sign in as a family member. I remember so clearly, the man told me, "Only family members," and I said, "I am the only family she has here," and he said, "Well, then why didn't you say you are family?" discreetly educating me on the procedure.

It was kind of upsetting to me that I had been forced into a mistruth (and, let's be honest; the idea that the accident of DNA should determine who is allowed access to you when you are dying in the hospital is ridiculously arbitrary), but I got over it.

Bumping the Bed

When I got up to her room, having gotten maybe an hour of sleep and determined to stay up all night with her so she wouldn't feel so alone, I felt like I had run some kind of gauntlet.

As I went to kiss her cheek in greeting, however, I accidentally bumped her bed, and it must have hurt her terribly because she bit my head off and I burst into tears. I was doing my very best to love her by alleviating pain and discomfort, and yet I had accidentally caused her even more pain.

I always think back to this incident in reference to relationships. We often "bump the bed" when we are trying to love others. We accidentally jar a wound and agony results when we are sincerely trying to make things better.

Diane always talked glowingly about all her friends from church and how wonderful they were, but I was not at all impressed. And eventually I realized it was mostly bravado on her part. I would stay eight to twelve hours a day and no one thought to feed me or come to relieve me long enough that I could take a bathroom break. Sometimes I didn't go to the bathroom for the whole eight to twelve hours I was there.

I think the boyfriend brought food twice. In sixty days.

I hated to leave her at the end of every day, but I realized that if I did not sleep, I would not be able to care for her at all.

When her friends did come, they mostly came to bring some gift, do a little song and dance, and then scurry away back into the light just as fast as they could (I know, I know. I did the same thing on that first day, but I pressed on and got better).

Or they stayed for hours obliging her to stay awake and engage when she had no strength to do so. Diane felt obligated to entertain them. They weren't caregiving. They were taking. I don't think they meant to. They just didn't reflect very deeply. Lack of experience and lack of reflection.

So, when I went back to Georgetown, I was worried that no one was caring for her. I called every day trying to reach someone to find out whether she was being adequately cared for. I asked her if she wanted me to come back and stay with her and she wouldn't answer me.

People would ask her if she needed anything and she would say, "No."

I gradually realized this was because nobody wants to have to ask someone to come stay by their side when they are dying. Least of all the child of missionaries who was weaned on the milk of self-sacrifice and that supreme principle of so many women—to never inconvenience anyone with their own needs.

I felt that people were willfully blind to what she needed. They asked and were only too happy to believe her when she said she didn't need them and gave them the out they wanted.

She was waiting for someone to care for her because they loved her, and not because they felt obligated to.

The Gift of Helps and Strategic Obtuseness

It offended me that people kept telling me I had what Christians call "the gift of helps"—a phrase I came to resent, as it often felt like a pass for others to opt out.

I did not feel I had any such gift. I felt I simply did what love calls for. Love calls us to roll up our sleeves and do what needs doing.

I wasn't a mother either, but I had eyes in my head. And some older friends who had witnessed my childhood speculated that being the oldest child of a blind mother gave me some caregiving insight others lacked.

I felt that others said I had the gift of helps so they could also imply that they themselves did not have that particular gift and thus excuse themselves from getting involved.

It took about ten years for me to realize I do kind of have a gift for sitting with others in the darkness that is, in fact, pretty rare.

I didn't see it then, but I am very comfortable in the Shadow of Death. I am comfortable in the presence of suffering. I am almost drawn to it, perhaps the way nurses and doctors are drawn to physical suffering.

They feel a calling to tend to people in their suffering. So, do I. I feel called to sit with people in the dark.

I know what it is to sit in the darkness alone and feel that it will suck all the light out of your soul. I don't want that for others.

Diane had a Japanese friend who went to high school with her in Belgium. She flew out to see Diane. I admired how she was able to make Diane laugh.

She was getting married in a week or two and Diane was supposed to be her maid of honor. She had met me once before, about six years earlier in Japan, but we were not really friends. Nevertheless, she asked me to be her maid of honor in Diane's place, back in the DC area.

I felt that was a pretty big ask, especially given that I cried all the time.

But I agreed, for Diane's sake.

If You See Something, Say Something

Before I left to go back to DC, I noticed that the whites of Diane's eyes had become greenish. I asked the nurse about it, and she winced and said, "That's because the cancer has gotten to her liver."

Trusting that the professionals had everything well in hand, I said no more, but called her parents on my way back to Chicago to let them know about this development.

The only formal-ish dress I had was black and after checking with Shihoko that it was ok, I wore that to the wedding.

I was so proud of myself. I got all the way through the wedding, made it all the way down the aisle at the end without crying, and then turned to the outside wall of the chapel when I got through the doors and gushed my usual firehose of agony.

The best man was very kind and gave me his handkerchief.

I would soon learn that while I was walking down that aisle at the end of that wedding, Diane was being wheeled down the hospital hallways and rushed into emergency surgery because that greenishness in the whites of her eyes was actually the result of a massive infection.

Do not "trust" that everyone is on top of everything. If you see something, say something. There are so many patients with so many symptoms for the healthcare professionals to stay on top of. Your eyes are helpful. Ask questions. Ask for help.

In this surgery, they had to open her back up. That wound never closed. She was buried with a ghastly, open wound, several inches deep and about seven inches long, from navel to sternum.

It became the metaphor for my life for the next two decades. It was like I toppled from a cliff and fell into that wound. The great chasm in her body was a chasm in the Valley of the Shadow of Death and it swallowed me whole.

Dropping Everything to Go and Die with My Beloved Friend

After two weeks in DC, it became clear to me that I needed to return to Chicago. Getting her to tell me whether she wanted me to come or not was like pulling teeth. She again could not ask for what she wanted. I was beginning to understand this, but I made her articulate that she would be happier with me there. I was, after all, taking incompletes in all my classes to go be with her. I wanted to make sure I wasn't going to be superfluous or unwanted.

My Skokie friends were kind enough to let me stay with them again. After I got there, Diane kept saying to me, "I feel like you are saving my life." By which she was also saying that she felt those nearest her had abandoned her to die. That is also how I knew she was in denial about how much time she had left.

I sang to Diane almost constantly. I guess it was the only way I knew to offer comfort to us both. I video recorded most of her waking hours and that got on people's nerves. Someone asked her how she felt about it, and she said she thought it might bother her if she didn't know how very much I loved her.

I hadn't seen her for most of the last twelve years, and I didn't want to lose a single moment of these last few precious hours of her life. I was also very protective of her energy and people thought I was too much of a fierce mother bear. I thought they were much too oblivious to her needs and her situation.

I remember one friend of hers complaining about Diane being irritable and my having to say, "You do realize she is never going to marry, have children, complete her degree, fulfill her felt mission in South Africa, everything is coming to an end."

I don't think she did. I don't think she had even let herself realize that Diane was dying, and soon. She actually let her own hurt feelings, so trivial under the circumstances, take center stage.

Sometimes dire circumstances bring out the best in people, but I think equally often they bring out the worst. It's the kind of pressure that reveals what's in your character.

James Allen, in *As a Man Thinketh*, writes, "Circumstances don't make the man. They reveal him."

I would modify that assertion. I think that our experiences simultaneously shape and reveal us. But the shaping is under our direction. We get to use experiences as a tool to shape our own character.

And when circumstances reveal some imperfection yet to be rectified, we need not feel shame. The circumstance has done us a favor by revealing where we are now, which helps us plot a course for where we want to go, who we want to become.

I'm sure each of us learned more from our experience with Diane about how to be in the presence of the shadow of death.

10

— · —

NOT UNTIL CHECK OUT TIME

What is the value of a life cut off in its prime? What is the point of living if you only have a few months or weeks or days left? What is the value and point of one moment of your life?

Normally, these are questions you ask when you receive your own terminal diagnosis. Unless, of course, you have been down this road before with a loved one, as I have (and maybe you have, too).

When you care for someone as they die young, you wrestle with all these questions vicariously and do yourself the favor of unraveling some of these existential riddles ahead of time.

That's how it worked for me. When I was diagnosed with Stage IV cancer, I recalled everything I had learned from Diane's experience, and I didn't have to come up with new answers to questions I was already satisfied with.

Allow me to share some of that with you.

Just Because Your Number's Up, Doesn't Mean It's Check Out Time

June 13, 2020

When my sweet friend died of stomach cancer, she had just turned thirty. Though she had returned to the States brittle and bruised by the brutal death of her mother, her heart chewed up with grief, in time, she began to heal. Her own cherry blossom season came round again, and she bloomed, loveliest of them all. In the last couple of years before she died, she was the happiest I had seen her in years. How wonderful that she achieved this renaissance before she died. Some people never do.

She was so full of life. She loved people, she loved God, she loved dancing, she loved poetry and song and learning, she loved nature. She just so loved being alive! And when she was diagnosed with stomach cancer, she fought hard. She fought for her life the way a mockingbird fights for her family — with no sense of proportion, no acknowledgement of the grossly superior size of her foe, focused only on what she has to lose. And she lived almost two years in that denial, thinking it was going to go away. But stomach cancer? I was amazed that she lasted as long as she did.

And now here she lay, emaciated, with almost no hair, and the life seemingly draining out of her onto the sheets into the bed, the floor, the ground, deep into the bowels of mother earth. And yet she still imagined, right up until a few weeks before she died, she was going to get better.

Her mother had died of breast cancer five years earlier. Her father was also in denial. I don't know what her boyfriend's understanding was, but he was certainly not helpful. Everyone else balking at the job, it fell to me to be the one to make her understand that she was dying.

Of course, I thought for a long time about how to do that. Finally, one day, sitting by her bed and looking into her eyes, I said, "How did your mother die?" (with the emphasis on the word *mother*, so she wouldn't miss the message). "Did she die like a saint?" And of course, she did. She was a missionary. It was kind of in the job description.

The Dawning and the Dimming and the Dawning Again

There was so much work to be done. And I tried to show her the relationships she needed to take care of before she reached her last day. I talked about her relationships with her father and her brother and how she needed to tie those up. She said, "Wow, I have so much work to do." She took it surprisingly well. At first.

And then, as the news sank in over the following days, she just checked out. She would not engage, and she pretended like she wasn't conscious for several days. She just gave up. She detached herself emotionally. Apparently, if you're not going to live a long time, acting alive is pointless. I understood her despair, but I didn't want her to lose her final days.

So, one day I pulled my chair up close and drew my face near to hers and we had a little heart to heart. I was always her big sister. And her mother was already gone, so it fell to me to be her touchstone of truth.

Standing there every day for two months, I spent so much time brooding and reflecting and grappling with this awful collision of Diane's youth and her death.

What is the value of a life cut off in its prime? Is this short life somehow less valuable than one that reaches the seventy-year mark?

I suppose it depends on what you think the purpose of a life is. What is the objective? Diane's motivating purpose was to go back to South Africa and continue serving homeless street girls in Cape Town. She had only been able to do that for four years before she had to go care for her mother in Johannesburg.

Just four years of her stated purpose. Was that valuable enough? Did she contribute enough to the world? Of course, we could write about all the other lovely things she did on this earth, all the people she loved and cared for, all the joy she gave to others through her dancing, the little girls she loved in the orphanage in South Africa, the child who died in her arms before she could get him to ER, her sweet little exchanges with Reverend Tutu.

Would that then be the sum of her purpose and her value?

Are Short Lives Less Meaningful Than Long Ones?

Is your life defective or incomplete if it doesn't endure for seventy or eighty years? Or if you didn't marry or have children, earn a degree, reach your career goals, get your name in the history books, save a life, or any other milestone of achievement you think is an essential element of a "full" life? What makes your life worthwhile? What is the point of you? What is the point of us?

I believe its value depends on its purpose. You don't have to believe in God or a higher being to believe in purpose. The human being is a meaning-making machine. Nobody can decide for you what your purpose is, and I am certainly not trying to peddle mine (though you are welcome to it, if it serves you). But I searched my heart over the course of those months. I realized what Diane and I both felt was the purpose of our lives (and I stand by it now, even though many other things about my worldview have changed).

I asked her, "Dear girl, what is the purpose of our life? Is it not to love others and to experience their love, and to love the divine and experience the love of the divine? And if so, that is something that you can do in seventy years, or seven years, or seven days, or seven minutes."

"And if that is the case, my love," I told her, "and you have even seven minutes left, your purpose is still valid." (I looked sternly into her watchful blue eyes, peeking up at me from beneath her wrinkled brow). "You do not get to check out, my love, until CHECK OUT TIME."

And you know what? She came back to us and rejoined the living for as long as she had left. She loved us. She let us love her. And I know she had her own loving exchange with the divine, always flowing back and forth like the breath that was still moving in her, no less mysterious on her last day than on her first. I think this was the most important lesson of my life, preparing me for my own future tango with death.

Life is not beautiful because it is long, my dear ones. It is beautiful because it is deep and full of love, full of joy, full of grace, and full of light.

Yes, I will keep chanting this to you until it flows naturally out of your own souls and one day you realize you are absolutely not afraid...

True Hope Must Be Valid Even If You Die
Saturday, June 13, 2020

How can I get you to appreciate the concept that our hope should never be in a particular outcome? Of course, we have a survival instinct built into our DNA and we wish to extend this to those we love as well; it's like a sympathetic survival instinct. And you are extending it to me because you love me, and for this, I am deeply grateful. I love you, too. Infinitely.

But perhaps it would be useful to make a distinction between hope and wishfulness or desire. We wish for certain outcomes. We wish for beauty, and not ugliness. We wish for love, and not loneliness. We wish to have pleasure and comfort and not suffering. We wish to live, and not die. These are our preferences. Our druthers. But you may have noticed, as I have, that with alarming frequency, we do not get our druthers.

Of what value is a hope that depends entirely upon your desired circumstance coming to pass? In my mind, peace is an inextricable element of hope. And peace must persist whether we get one outcome or another. I do not see how you can have peace if your hope depends upon something that is uncertain. These ideas are antithetical. I mean, since we know that life is always uncertain, I don't see how a hope like that could even exist. I believe that hope and peace must both live outside of our circumstances.

At some point I think that words like *faith* and *hope* and *peace* and *joy* are all really just shades of perfect love (the way white light can be broken down into individual colors). The more you focus on them and what they mean, the more their definitions begin to merge into each other right there in the center of perfect love.

So, let's talk about faith. I do not believe that faith means you believe the thing you want is going to come to pass. Or I do not put much stock in that kind of faith. Such faith is fragile and fickle, frail. Moreover, that kind of faith is immediately and inevitably destroyed when the outcome you end up with is not the one you desired. What possible value could there be in a faith that is so easily shattered?

I believe that true hope and true faith entail a deep knowledge that no matter what happens, you will be ok. Even if you die.

Won't You Be Ok?

I never noticed this about the way we use *You won't die*, or *It won't be the end of the world*, as assurances that anything is survivable, until this month when I started contemplating my own potentially imminent death. Because what we are also saying when we use those expressions is that if death happens, we will not be ok. Almost everything is survivable. Except death. It seems that death is the one thing we do fear. It is the worst possible scenario. If death happens, well, in that case, no, you will not be ok.

Won't you? The fact of my having lived will exist for eternity. Nothing will ever change that fact. And I wish to be a voice always singing in the back of your mind,

Life is not beautiful because it is long, my loves, but because it is deep and full of love, full of joy, full of grace, and full of light, all of these flowing in and flowing out like the tides.

It's ok if life is short.

If my life comes to an "early" end, it does not mean death won, and I lost. I can win and still come to the completion of my life sooner than we had wanted. You don't win by extending or determining the number of your days. You win by not letting the number of your days determine how you live and by savoring and appreciating each one. You win by making sure everyone you love knows in their bones how deeply you love them before you go. You win by weaseling your way into the hearts of those souls you adore and dwelling within them long after you are gone.

You can win the fight by how you spend your life and how lovingly, beautifully, peacefully you die. Death is part of life; it is not to be feared. And if you live it meaningfully throughout, you are less likely to die feeling your life is unfinished.

I am happy with the life I have lived. I am happy with who I am. I have very few regrets. I have spent my whole life loving people hard and trying to bring them healing. That's what I wanted to do.

Yes, dears, I want to live, and I will fight this cancer like a honey badger, as long as there is reason to believe those efforts are not futile. I do not want to leave you with holes in your lives. I'd like to keep on loving you for many years, making you laugh, sometimes making you cry, hopefully making you think about things that matter... enriching you in any way that I might, and being enriched by you, too.

But at the end of the day and at the end of my days, true hope means:

Everything is going to be ok, my loves.

Even if I die.

11

— • —

WALKING HER HOME AS FAR AS I COULD

I'm not sure what causes denial. I think we all experience different kinds of denial in different circumstances. I don't know if it's bravery that makes us forge ahead with our eyes open, refusing to acknowledge the pain, or if it's some kind of stupidity or something we just have no control over whatsoever.

I am thankful that I did not have the luxury of denial about Diane's dying, because I think it empowered me to be present with my friend through the worst of her experience.

As for my own suffering... well, that's another story for another chapter. Let me just admit that it turns out that I am by no means immune to denial.

Every day I was exhausted. I always felt bad going home to my friend's house to sleep, but I knew that if I didn't rest, I wouldn't be able to keep caring for her in this way.

One day I had slept in a little before going to the hospital to try to catch up on my rest just a little, and that day, of course, was the one day she was in terrible pain and was calling out my name and I wasn't there. So, I never did that again.

I just prayed fervently that she would not die while I was away at night. That she would wait for me, so I could walk with her to the end of that path.

Last Chance - Losing Diane's Mind

While Diane was still in the hospital, before they moved her to hospice, they were going to give her an epidural so that she could be in less pain but still be conscious and able to enjoy her loved ones. The Fentanyl caused her to hallucinate while she was talking, and it was impossible to have a conversation. (As I've mentioned, the poor girl didn't eat for the last sixty days of her life, and she kept hallucinating food floating in the air that she would reach out and try to pluck and eat). She wasn't with us most of the time, even when she was awake.

That day, waiting for the surgery, was one of the longest of my life. The procedure kept being postponed for hours at a time because her blood was too thin, and they were trying to fix that.

The waiting and the fits and starts reminded me of the chaotic period following my little brother's death in 1971, when I was four. We were going to fly from our home in Kansas to New York, to be with my father's family, to grieve there, in their presence. I think my father had just stopped functioning. My parents had simply collapsed emotionally, and our family was imploding.

I was nervous about the plane trip and a grandmother who was a little scary because I didn't know her, so I was trying to gear myself up for this challenge, but I didn't know when this was going to happen, and it kept getting postponed. Screw up your energy for something painful and scary, have the goal post moved, wait in limbo, lose the courage you had mustered. Rinse and repeat. It was utterly exhausting.

I was four, but I remember thinking I couldn't even depend on the things I was afraid of. Everything was shifting sand.

All my hope was fixed on this procedure for Diane because without it, essentially, we had already lost her. She simply wasn't present anymore. I walked beside the gurney as they rolled her down to the OR. Her father, the boyfriend and I sat tensely but tiredly in the waiting area, and after a while two residents, a man and a woman, came out and sat down and talked with us.

They were not going to be able to do the procedure. Ever.

I cried like it was the end of the world. It was the end of Diane.

They were so compassionate. They just sat with us while I cried.

It is odd. I was the only one crying. I'm not sure the others were really allowing themselves to process what this meant. I often had the feeling I was the only person in Diane's whole sphere of relationships who had her eyes open. Other than her surgeon and the other health care professionals, perhaps I was.

I don't know how much of that was because I already knew the way—and how much was because my particular experience and constitution had somehow equipped me not to be afraid of the dark.

But I will also say this: we needed a guide. And there was no one guiding us through our grief.

Hospice

Shortly thereafter, Diane began to decline. One day, they loaded her into an ambulance and drove her across the parking lot to the hospice facility. We moved her in.

It was so much more peaceful than the hospital, with its constant noise and activity. There is no real rest in a hospital. Hospice still wasn't home, but her wound required too much care for us to manage on our own. This was the next best option.

The nurses and doctors couldn't understand why she was still alive. They said old people die slowly—young people crash. But Diane died like a leaf floating downward in the wind. Slowly. Gently. Stubbornly. She just wanted to live. She was so attached to life.

We began to wonder if she didn't feel closure. She had always longed to marry. So, we arranged a kind of ceremony for her and her boyfriend—a time for them to declare their love for each other. Still, she hung on. We thought maybe she wasn't sure we were going to be ok.

Be Thou My Vision

Be Thou My Vision was always my favorite hymn, as it was Diane's, no doubt not only because it is beautiful, but because we both happened to have blind mothers. It was one of the reasons we were introduced to each other by mutual friends. I had never met anyone else who had a blind mother, and it was definitely a powerful bonding element.

One day when she was in hospice, she had already kind of gone into a semi-coma and was barely conscious most of the time. A nurse accidentally gave her an overdose of Benadryl because the company had changed the strength of the medicine without changing the appearance of the packaging. And she went into a seizure where she was blind and very afraid, which is something that had happened to her mother during her illness and was one of the things Diane had been dreading all this time.

So, I went behind the bed and put my hands gently on her shoulders and I just sang *Be Thou My Vision*.

Be Thou My Vision, oh Lord of my heart
Naught be all else to me save that Thou art
Thou my best thought by day or by night.
Waking or sleeping, Thy presence my light.

I sang until she came out of the seizure. It was one of our precious moments and seemed to give a lot of comfort to her stepmom and dad at the same time (her stepmother said it sounded like there was an angel in the room).

The nurse happened to be Japanese, and she was at least as traumatized by the event and her involvement as the rest of us were. It was a grace to me that I was able to tell her in Japanese (not because she didn't speak English perfectly well, but because it enabled us to have a private conversation in a room full of people) to please not worry. It wasn't her fault, no one was angry with her, everything was going to be ok.

Looking back, I guess I felt that it was usually my job to manage the peace quotient in the room, to soothe all the hearts involved so we would all have a smoother journey. (I remember trying to do this on the day that Brian died and failing. Perhaps I have been trying to edit that day ever after.)

Flash Resurrection

They gave Diane an antidote for the Benadryl overdose, and the most astonishing thing happened. She woke up and was perfectly clear and conscious, like she hadn't been for weeks. She sat up in bed, and it was like she was holding court. It was a temporary resurrection.

We all sat around the bed, and she spoke French with her father, and she told stories and laughed and we asked questions.

It was this little miracle that we had her back for a few hours. The palliative care doctors (two lovely women Diane had previously regarded with antipathy as the angels of death because they would come by to visit while she was still in the hospital to talk to her about going to hospice) looked at each other in surprise and said they saw a clinical trial coming out of that.

And then she pretty quickly returned to the same state she had been in. And she was in what I would call a full coma for the last three days of her life.

Singing Her into the Light

On Father's Day, a lot of friends came over in the morning, and we sat around and laughed and told stories about our memories with Diane and I think she decided we were going to be ok, after all.

Her brother David had a private (one-sided) conversation with her and said his goodbyes and went back to Minnesota.

I read a letter to her about how much I loved her and what I thought about the afterlife and just saying goodbye.

One by one, everyone said their goodbyes and went home.

I have heard that women often won't die in front of their families, in front of their husbands or children. When Diane's dad and stepmother went for a walk, it was just Dave (the boyfriend) and me. And something about her breathing changed.

So, Dave went to get the nurse and when she came back, she said, "Elisa, sing that song you always sing to her."

Well, I sang every song I knew to her, but I often sang her favorite song from the Psalms, so I sang it then.

The Lord is my light and my salvation
The Lord is the strength of my life.
The Lord is my light and my salvation
The Lord is the strength of my life.
And I will not be afraid, no I will not be afraid.
The Lord is my light, the Lord is my light, the Lord is my light.
And then a couple of lines from the Psalms via John Michael Talbot,
I was glad when they said unto me,
Let us go to the house of the Lord
And now my feet are standing within
your gates, Jerusalem.

And as I finished, she took her last breath.
It was as if I sang her into His gates.
That was one of the most sacred gifts of my life.

I was unspeakably grateful to be able to do that.

I don't know if I have ever done anything I felt was more important with my life.

Grieving Alone (Again)

When my brother Brian died, my parents grieved in secret. They grieved at night behind closed doors. I think their pain was too raw, too intimate, too devastating to expose to the eyes of others.

As a result, there were people who actually said my mother didn't care about her little boy because they didn't see her cry.

Unfortunately, I didn't see my parents cry either. So, I felt that I was completely alone in this horrible place of unexpressed grief. I wrapped up this wounded piece of my soul in a shroud of unconsciousness and buried it deep in my psyche.

I didn't know any of these people in Diane's sphere in Chicago, except her immediate family, who weren't there very much. And the family I was staying with did not know Diane.

So, after she passed, I had no one to call. I did call a couple of her friends and recounted the details of her passing, but they were not people I had a connection with.

Once Diane was gone, I felt utterly alone.

And when I went back to DC, no one there had known her. So, I felt that I was completely alone in my grief again, and this time, I was developmentally able to grieve.

I was over developmentally able to grieve.

And thus, I sobbed for seven years.

My tears were a river of pain, and I just wanted to float away on them and let them carry me out to sea and drown me.

12

— · —

AGAIN!

How tired are you of the glass half empty metaphor?

My favorite pandemic meme was a picture of a glass of yellow liquid that said, "When you realize it doesn't matter whether it's half empty or half full, it's a glass of pee!"

Well, that's an apt metaphor for the topic at hand.

And yet—there is hope here...

Measuring the Air in the Glass and Not the Water

What gets you out of bed in the morning?

I have often felt like Martin Luther, who may have been bipolar, and who allegedly said, "Most days I am so depressed I can't even get out of bed."[1] I can empathize. I have spent years of my life in that place.

Perhaps you have been there too. Perhaps this diagnosis of cancer or some other illness or grief has put you there. What do you have to be awake to?

To be sure, a great deal of this may be chemical or wound based and that needs to be dealt with. But so often we attribute mild depression to circumstance, when in fact it is more about focus.

Our outlook and enjoyment of life has so much more to do with focus than circumstance.

When you see the glass "half empty" you are really measuring the air, the lack, the deprivation.

Half of perception is focus. You can focus on the air in the glass as the absence of water or you can focus on the presence of the water.

Why do our minds and memories seem to privilege pain?

I am a four on the Enneagram and we fours are very attached to our pain. In fact, we pretty much define ourselves by our pain. We are not only comfortable sitting in the dark, we generally prefer it. And we tend to drive others crazy with our tendency to dwell deep and dark so much of the time.

Fours generally believe there is something fundamentally flawed about themselves, and they get so overwhelmed by their emotions that they often tend towards suicide.

Sylvia Plath was a four. She is one who didn't make it. She had to end her life to end her pain.

I almost didn't make it. I wanted to die so many times.

For at least the first twenty years of my life, I could see almost exclusively the agony and misfortune of my childhood. The story I told was tragic and in it I was a victim of all kinds of wrong.

To be fair, I really did have more than the usual allotment of adversity for an American (my ACE, Adverse Childhood Experience, score is almost a 10 out of 10. When I add traumas not included in the survey, I feel like it comes to about 16).

However, there was also a lot of love, joy, strength, and beauty in my childhood that, for much too long, I allowed to be totally overshadowed by the dark stuff.

And yet that early adversity is also precisely the reason I was able to rise out of later darkness and into the light.

So many people say, "There is no point in digging up the past."

I do not agree that we should never examine the past. There is very definitely a time to dig up the past and that is when a part of your soul has been buried alive, as mine had been since early childhood.

Once healing has taken place, however, as I posted on one of my many blogs in 2019:

It behooves us greatly to re-write every painful memory to include the joy and beauty in and around those moments. Why should we let pain out scream the sweeter emotions that also ran in the swift flowing current of our tumultuous lives? Preserve the joy and beauty! Don't let them float in our memories as something less substantial than our suffering! Don't let them be the ephemeral foam and froth, the waves that take shape and then dissolve. Let them be the lovely stones and the hard gleaming surfaces indelibly written upon by the waves! And as you heal, let pain wash away with the waves.

Countering the Negativity Bias

Many people respond to the pain in their lives by trying to numb out.

For some people, the odious term "to kill time" is about fleeing from the "pain" of boredom.

Others kill time with more passion. They are trying to deaden their own nerves so they might not feel the agony of their lives. They are trying to anesthetize. Whether through alcohol, drugs, food, extreme sports, workaholism, Netflix...

The first time I asked this question about why our minds privilege pain, I had not yet encountered the idea of the negativity bias.[2]

Well, now I know that it wasn't just part of my inherently flawed personality. Human beings are hard-wired to remember and react to negative events. It's part of how our brains have kept us safe for zillions of years. We remember those things that were life-threatening because those things are essential in staying alive. A beautiful day is not so important to remember as it has less to offer in the way of tangible life-preservation merit.

Trauma stays with us forever because our minds don't want us to ever repeat that experience. Historically, our brain used it to protect us, but it is questionable how much we need it now.

It is true. The brain you were issued at birth may have been pre-formatted to work this way. But guess what? We now know about the miracle of neuroplasticity. You can rewire it! You can do a factory reset! Well, ok—it's not quite as instantaneous as pushing the little red button on the bottom of your garbage disposal, but you can reformat and rewire your brain.

You can absolutely choose to spend more time remembering and savoring the positive experiences in your life and give them more stage time than the other stuff.

Let me be clear, you must do the hard work of healing first. After that you can rewire your brain for a healthy positivity.

Two things about the following poem. First, I wrote it for myself, not for the world, as a reminder to wake the hell up. I share it with you because it is part of my story. It is also a bit of an outraged love song to presence, a reminder that our time here is precious.

It is not a judgment against those who must sometimes step away from life to heal, to endure, or simply to survive (as I have many times). I would say that taking time out is not at all the same as killing time. There are moments when retreat is a form of courage too.

May these words be an invitation, not a burden—an offering of light, not a demand.

Redeem the Time
Resolve in yourself
that you will never again
speak of killing time.
Time is just another word for life,
a measurement of quantity.
To kill time is tantamount to
suicide with a small s.
Killing yourself for stretches of time
by choosing to be absent,
dead to yourself,
dead to those you are closest to,
dead to the world,
perhaps dead to God.
Just dead.
Betimes.
In the in-between times.
While you yet have breath in you!!!
Why would you do that???
How many micro suicides might you avoid
by committing to be ever and always
redeeming the time?

On the Savoring of Moments...

Wednesday, May 27, 2020

Someone has said (it is often attributed to Cesare Pavese), "We don't remember days, only moments," but need this be so, especially for the wordsmith!? How many moments in a single day might we immortalize by merely clothing them in the splendor of language?

This is the glory of writing! That you may take the ephemeral and clothe it with an inky substance that, applied to the concrete and blissfully tangible, touchable, smellable page, endures beyond the power of one's otherwise relatively feeble mental repository.

It occurs to me that there are hundreds, if not thousands, of days I don't remember. It grieves me to count my losses. Surely each of them had tens if not hundreds of moments worthy of reflection in the years that would follow. And I let so many of them slip away, never to be retrieved.

I wish someone had made this truth known to me in my youth. I would have done three things.

(I mean I probably would not have unless, perhaps, it had been three really persuasive ghosts named after verb tenses—the ghost of Elisa present and her extracontemporary companions...)[3]

First, I would have savored moments like expensive chocolates, like rare perfumes. I would have become a collector and a connoisseur of moments!

Second, I would have carefully curated my memories such that the ecstasies and the everyday joys might at least balance, if not outweigh, the heavy emotional burden of the moments of agony and malaise that seem so often to eclipse my happier memories.

Third, where the beautiful memories were shared, I would have striven to help the other souls about me capture those memories for their own private collections. I would have brought them often to their minds that these thoughts might remain alive.

I am thinking of Oliver Wendell Holmes, Jr., referring to words as the skins of living thoughts[4], and I am thinking of thoughts as the translations of moments.

When I first wrote this, I was also thinking that I had perhaps as much life ahead of me as I had behind me [Ah. Would that it were so, dear self] and, as there is no time like the present (and, according to Eckhart Tolle, no time but the present), I hereby resolve to pursue these three lofty goals of savoring, curating, and sharing the lovely moments that comprise this beautiful life I am living — through the magnificent gift of language!

Diane's Last Chapter—a Painful Mixture of the Holy and the Horrific

It is hard for me to imagine a more excruciating existence than Diane's last weeks of life. I believe you would literally have to refer to the lives of torture victims and martyrs to find suffering that exceeded hers. The nasal-gastric tube was bad enough. Being constantly hungry and dreaming of food and not being able to consume anything but grapefruit juice for sixty days is pretty hellish. But to have a seven-inch incision down the middle of your person, three to four inches deep that won't close, and which has to be opened and cleaned and re-dressed four times a day, I can't personally imagine much worse. You would have to go to a Stephen King novel or *Foxe's Book of Martyrs*.

I have a fairly weak stomach when it comes to seeing other people's wounds, and this was kind of the mother of all wounds as far as I was concerned, so for the first week or two I would sit in the corner and hide behind my laptop when they would change the wound and try very hard not to see anything. But gradually I got acclimated and sometimes I would go and hold her hand while they changed it.

i thank you god

One day when they were changing that ghastly wound, I stood beside her and held her hand and she asked me to talk about my dissertation so she could fall asleep. Not to worry, being stout of heart, I was not offended. I thought, *Only because you are dying, am I going to let that pass and pretend that you did not just imply that my life's passion is your go-to treatment for insomnia.* As we were both English majors and lovers of poetry, I just grinned and said, "Why don't I tell you a poem instead?" When she assented, we invited the holy into the horrific, and I recited from memory ee cummings's poem *"i thank You God for most this amazing day."*[5]

It is a poem that does what only the best poetry can do: it insists on wonder in the face of mortality. It praises trees and sky and breath and sensation itself, declaring existence—not despite suffering, but within it—to be an extravagant yes. It speaks in the voice of someone who knows what it is to die and yet wakes up astonished to be alive again, senses sharpened, eyes and ears newly opened to the sheer gift of being.

As I came to the end of the poem, her eyes were closed, and I thought that she had fallen asleep, and I had done my job. But as I finished the last line, her eyes popped open and she cried, "Again!" with so much enthusiasm my heart thrilled.

And so, of course, I recited it a second time. Once she had decided that she would not check out until checkout time, she went on sucking the nectar out of every moment that she had. She was so in love with life, and she drank it to its very dregs.

Our Last Adventure

October 6, 2020

One day when she could still walk some, I helped her get dressed up in overalls and we took down all her bags of fluids and tubes from her IV pole and stuffed them in her pockets and snuck her out of the hospital in a wheelchair (yes, I just said *snuck*). I was so nervous as I pulled up the car to get her, I felt like I was robbing a bank! We just drove five minutes to my friend's house, where we sat down and had a popsicle on the couch, laughing about our little crime spree.

It was our last adventure. But we seized that day and found a way to infuse it with joy amidst the pain. She was so in love with life.

And I thought of how much life seems to be wasted on people who are not in love with it, who can carelessly speak of "killing time." And I resolved that I would never again speak of killing time, for time is just another word for life, and it does not come to us in an infinite supply.

After Diane died, I cried for years. But I sought healing and found it in time.

The cherry blossoms came around again.

The poet Mary Oliver asks, "What will you do with your one wild and precious life?" [6] Will you give yourself in service to others? Will you dance, will you laugh, will you sneak out of the hospital to have a popsicle on the couch? Or will you turn sourly inside yourself and shut out the precious gift of life you are yet in possession of?

I almost let my grief extinguish my joy. But I decided to follow Diane's example to love life and live it to its very dregs. And if I could have just one prayer for you, my friends, it is this: that every morning when you wake up you, too, would open your eyes wide and like Diane, cry with all the fervor that is in you, "Again!"

I printed this in a large, beautiful font and posted it beside my bed, "Again!"

Please feel free to take this as your rallying cry, too. Seize each day anew and again.[7]

---

1. *Luther.* Directed by Eric Till, performance by Joseph Fiennes, MGM Home Entertainment, 2004.

2. Gilmartin, Brianna. *"What Is the Negativity Bias?" Verywell Mind*, 11 Apr. 2019, http://www.verywellmind.com/negative-bias-4589618 .

3. What?? You take exception to extracontemporary? I am a linguist! What is the point of me if not to occasionally bring lexical offerings to my fellow speakers of our mother tongue?

4. Holmes, Oliver Wendell, Jr. *Towne v. Eisner*, 245 U.S. 418, 425 (1918).

5. Cummings, E. E. *Complete Poems, 1904–1962.* Edited by George J. Firmage, Liveright, 1994.

6. Oliver, Mary. *New and Selected Poems.* Beacon Press, 1992.

7. I feel like this would make a beautiful tattoo.

13

— · —

SHIPWRECKED

Have you ever been shipwrecked? Even once? If not, may your luck continue, but I think at least one or two shipwrecks are pretty standard fare for the human biography.

I've been shipwrecked several times in my life, but this was the mother of all shipwrecks for me. It was actually the culmination of several shipwrecks.

My ship had been battered into bits, and I was floating in the debris, half drowned.

Sacred Objects

After Diane finally passed, I had time to think about my situation. We went over to her house, and I selected a few of her belongings to remember her by (as if her presence wasn't indelibly inscribed on my soul).

I was sad that she had not selected anything to bequeath to me specifically, to render it the more sacred. It's one of those things that her denial denied me.

I mostly selected things that I had given her over the years, and she had treasured: a green heart sweater of mine we took turns wearing in college, a cloth jewelry box I had given her for a birthday, a musical bunny/picture frame I had bought her in Tokyo where the stuffed bunny's arm turns as he cranks the music box.

I never did find the little crystal model of Sofia I had bought her in Istanbul. No matter where I traveled, I liked to bring her something.

Caregiving Scripts

While at the house, I noticed something quietly heartbreaking: I had taken pictures of everyone else with Diane, but none with her and me together.

I hadn't been thinking about myself in those moments, and, it seemed, no one else had either. Only later did I let myself feel the disappointment I had not had the luxury to feel while in the flow of caregiving, this piercing realization of being unseen in my role.

A couple of people brought me food, like twice, but no one thought to offer a break or check in. I'd come from DC to Chicago; I wasn't part of the church community or close friends with most of the people there, and in the absence of shared history, I slipped through the cracks.

That experience opened my eyes to the invisible labor of caregiving and how vital it is to have coordination, compassion, and someone watching out for the caregiver, too.

No one in this scenario seemed to have a script for how to care for someone—and for each other—in the final days of a life.

Her father, a missionary who had lost his wife in almost the same way just five years earlier, might have had one, but he didn't. Her pastors might have drawn from experience, but their congregation was made up mostly of young adults—few parents, and almost no one who seemed familiar with the rhythms and rituals of dying.

I had a deep acquaintance with grief, but I didn't have a script either. The hospital chaplain, whom we had hoped might guide us with some spiritual insight or practical wisdom, had little to offer.

No one stepped forward to take responsibility for orchestrating this sacred and supremely consequential passage. Somehow, by default more than design, I became "it."

The American Approach to Dying

The problem with what seems to me to be the dominant American approach to illness—fight it tooth and nail to the last breath and treat death as a failure—is that people often don't say the things they need to say or set their affairs in order. Nor do they even seem to think about how they want their last hour to go... or how they want to be remembered after they are gone.

Diane fought to the very last breath. You may find that admirable. I find it tragic.

Somehow, there has to be a balance. If you are fighting so hard that you lose your last days and hours with your loved ones, what have you gained?

The doctors kept saying to me, "Go back and live your life."

But some of those same healthcare professionals (the surgeon herself and a couple of the hospice nurses) also said after she was gone that they also had best friends who had died, and they wished they had done for their friends what I had done for mine.

9/11 (When Death Wrecks Your Life It Can Be Very Thorough)

I returned to grad school where no one knew Diane. No one had any idea what hell I had just been through. I lived alone and was not part of any spiritual community at that time. I continued crying constantly. Woke up crying, cried throughout the day, lay at home bawling until I cried myself to sleep—for a year.

In *For Whom the Bell Tolls*, Hemingway describes a young Belgian orderly in the Eleventh Brigade who, after losing all five friends from his village, continues serving meals while silently weeping.[1] His trauma is so deep that he cries throughout every meal, unable to suppress his grief. That has always been my touchstone image of PTSD tears, and that is how I cried much of the time.

I dreamed every night for one year that Diane was alive again just so I could watch her die again. It was always my responsibility. In the dreams, all the weight of her dying was on me.

I had no support system. I had just been abandoned by my closest Georgetown friend and, as is the way with the dynamics of schism, a whole cluster of "friends" went with her. I had put syntax, my least favorite linguistic subject, off till my very last class and I kept having to run out of class and cry convulsively in the hallway. I sat in class and tears silently streamed down my face. My professor (notably not a sociolinguist) did not give a rat's big toe. No one could understand why I was so affected by Diane's death. I was utterly alone in my grief.

Diane had died on Father's Day of 2001. I had returned to DC, broken into splinters. On September 11, I was an earwitness to the Pentagon attack. I was outside and heard the crash and saw the pillar of smoke rising from the wreck from a couple of miles away. It was all just par for the course. My life had blown up. It was like my lifequake was accompanied by a life tsunami. It was all perfectly poetic.

In the meantime, I consumed copious quantities of alcohol and prayed that God would take my life. I prayed off and on for at least seven years that God would just let me die. I felt utterly abandoned. The pain was too heavy to bear.

I worked like a crazy person. And I worked on my dissertation all the time, but I was just spinning my wheels. I think I wrote ten different dissertations and deleted them. I was let go by Georgetown several times and had to keep reapplying for mercy and reinstatement.

But allow me now to briefly skip ahead a couple of years to share a story out of order because it illustrates my long shipwreck. It took place in Korea in 2010, two years after my trauma therapy, when I was clearly still healing.

Pia, Proxy for My Most Problematic Ghosts

In 2010, I went to Korea for two years to teach English at a foreign language boarding high school, most reluctantly. Some more healing happened while I was in Korea, although my thyroid went crazy, and I gained a ton of weight and became very depressed. I drank profuse quantities of soju (which is forty to fifty proof alcohol).

One poignant experience in Korea rather epitomizes my whole decade of shipwreck and my lifelong affinity for any creature cowering in the shadow of death. We teachers lived in a small apartment building at the foot of a mountain. More wondrously, at the foot of that mountain, was a park featuring several huge burial mounds inside which were the tombs of ancient Korean kings and queens. The mounds are the size of small houses and shaped very like giant breasts.

I made my way that night through the mountainous cityscape between parked cars and rain ravaged buildings in Buk Jeong. Gushing torrents of rain washed over me, like a typhoon, one of those storms where the ocean seems to have climbed up into the sky with the express purpose of rushing back out of it to inundate the land in powerful, pounding vertical waves.

Over the years, I had found myself caught in rain like that in the Far East more times than I could now remember. Mother nature has never been more empathic than she was that night, however, gushing water from the sky as I gushed grief from my soul.

Staggering through the rain, I cried at least as torrentially behind my umbrella. Such a deafening, heavy rain does provide one benefit for a white foreigner in Asia, which is a rare moment of a degree of much longed-for privacy in public. In normal weather, you are watched everywhere you go, from the time you leave your home in the morning until you return to it in the evening. You are always on stage. There I was, a tall, middle-aged white woman sobbing like an abandoned child, deplorably reinforcing the Asian stereotypes about Americans and their childish, undisciplined displays of emotion. I was glad to be hidden beneath an umbrella, within a storm.

Dead Kitten in a Shoebox

With a dead kitten in a shoebox under my left arm, I awkwardly hung onto a tin cup with my right hand. At the same time, I struggled to wield an umbrella against the torrents, trying to shield the kitten with it more than myself. Between my tears and the rain, I was trying to see into the darkness through two panes of falling water. Anyone who saw me must have thought I had lost my mind. And I guess I had. For the evening. Just completely surrendered to the madness of grief.

I had been gone all day to Busan, where I had bought food and dishes for that tiny little scrap of a cat I had rescued. I was tutoring the little girl who had first introduced me to the kittens a month or two before. One day, my impish eleven-year-old student had dragged me out to survey the little feline colony again.

There were lots of cats of various sizes around, but to one side of a set of stairs that led up to a restaurant, I came across this pathetic creature, sitting on her haunches, breathing with great difficulty, looking as if she were already draped over death's patient lower jaw, just waiting for it to close.

Though there was activity all around her, she seemed to sit completely isolated in her suffering. The sidewalk was part of a fairly busy intersection, where she was ignored by passersby as though she were a pool of vomit or a pile of feces, edited out of their visual experience like so much of the unsightly refuse which is neither pleasant nor polite to notice. The smell was sickening, as the pestilent smell of death will be.

Knowing she couldn't have more than two weeks to live, but unable to ignore my inner Mother Teresa, I looked to see what I had that I might cart her home in. Finding nothing, I went back to my student's mother, holding the stinky little bag of fleas in my hands, and asked for a sack or a box.

I don't know if I can describe the look the mother gave me. Incredulity, disdain, horror? Disgust? I think with a mixture of confusion and pity, as though I were mentally ill, as though I were trying to save a maggot from a pile of decay and take it home with me for a pet.

She handed me a shopping bag, which I gratefully accepted. I put the kitten inside and rolled down the top of the bag a bit so I could control it better. I called her Pia, for the text abbreviation, Pain in the Ass (although with my flair for melodrama it could, in the end, have been short for *Pietà*), because she struggled so much for the hour and a half it took to bring her home on the train in a paper sack.

I found it unbelievable how much energy she had to fling herself around in there when she was already mostly dead. And she stank to high heaven. I stood apart from the other passengers so they wouldn't smell her and be more inclined to complain. Of course, it was against the rules to carry an animal on the train. I managed to keep a straight face and everyone else kindly managed to pretend they did not notice.

Kitty Hospice

I filled a bucket with warm water as soon as we got home and promptly plunged her into it. She was exactly as indignant and irate as I expected. I dried her off with a towel and let her stalk around as mad as she wished, complaining at the top of her tiny little lungs. The fact that she could do so was heartening.

She may have stayed by herself the first night. But she soon took to coming over by my large warm body as I lay on my futon on the floor and shortly took to climbing up and lying on top of me. The precious little ragged bundle of skin and bones and bits of fur had come to sit on my chest just at the base of my neck, purring up a storm, hour after hour, day after day. A premonition, perhaps, of the storm I would bury her in.

I think I was surprised she had come to love me. I had not counted on it. Of course, I already loved her, else I would not have brought her home and set up my makeshift kitty hospice. I couldn't let her suffer and die all loveless and alone on a dirty, back street in downtown Busan. But when she started showing so much improvement, I lost sight of the hospice mission.

That is why, on this Saturday, exactly one week after I had rescued her, I was so worried about her health, eager to get home and present the kitty accouterments I had procured and start the long process of fattening her up.

I threw down all my bags and clothes and took off my shoes and then stood, feeling sick at her stillness from the doorway. As I came all the way in and closed the door behind me, I saw her across the room, stretched out and still on the pillow where I had left her, already stiff and cold, a trail of feces on the pillow where her tiny bowels had apparently failed her at the moment of death.

The Shadow of Death, Again

I stood perfectly still in the entryway, stunned. It should not have been so very unexpected; I knew she was mostly dead when I found her. Yet, somehow, I was not prepared. Ice crept down my fingers and through my stomach. Such a tiny animal, but my whole apartment felt pregnant with death. And it wasn't just that death had come to her, but it had come on my watch, in my care, in my absence, in my neglect. I had left her, and it was as though she had died because I was not there. She had died completely alone.

I tried to collect my frozen thoughts. I had to bury her. I needed something to dig with. I didn't want to just put her in a shoebox without any padding. It was too cold and sterile and inhumane. I found an expensive fluffy hand towel that I had been given as a gift. I gently wrapped the kitten in the towel and put her in the box. I realized I had nothing to dig with. I ransacked my kitchen. I didn't think a spoon would be adequate. I found a tin measuring cup and a sturdy butter knife I thought might suffice. I put on some kind of rain jacket and my running shoes.

I staggered down the stairs, past the sweet dog who was imprisoned there in his five-foot sphere of cement that was his entire world. I staggered down the alley getting more and more soaked as I proceeded, through the alleys and side streets, around parked cars, until I reached the mouth of the mountain path. I took the more direct route up, not the sidewalk that ambled gradually along a slighter slope.

I took the steep slope where there was no real path at first, then a path with wooden boards placed horizontally as makeshift steps, something between steps and a ladder pressed into the earth. It was slippery and wet, and I was trying to see through my blubbering tears and the rain and the darkness and my umbrella and I had no way to balance myself with both arms full.

Wanting to Fling Myself Off the Mountain

The mountain seemed unforgiving as I fell on my knees against the cold soggy ground again and again—but I didn't drop my precious cargo. I felt that all the cumulative darkness of my life was sucking me in, and what I really wanted to do was just find a deep enough recess to fling myself into with the kitten in my arms and bury myself deep in the mud between the trees.

I had a flash memory of being four and crossing a street without having my three-year-old baby brother's hand, of his senseless, bloody death. I had also the constant presence of my intimate friend at whose bedside I stood for months while I watched her die her hellish death to stomach cancer for some 87,600 minutes, one grim, grueling minute at a time.

I reached the top of the lower level of the mountain. I looked for a spot that would be suitable, knowing it was almost certainly illegal to bury an animal here, though it occurred to me that an animal might die here without breaking any laws.

I found a place just off the path enough that it wouldn't draw attention, but open enough between the trunks of trees that I could carve a little grave. Although the ground was rain soaked, it was also clay-like and stony and almost impossible to dig in. I fumbled through, now using the tin cup, now my bare hand and fingernails, till I had culled what might serve as a very shallow grave, nowhere near big enough for the shoe box.

Wrapping her gently in the towel, I laid her limp little body tenderly in the ground and covered her as best I could. I was crying too hard to really concentrate on doing this well. I was afraid it would wear away in time. Either the earth would be washed away with rain, or some other combination of the elements and animals might uncover her, but it was the very most I had the strength for. And I hoped the softness of that luxury towel would somehow compensate for this otherwise cold and inadequate burial in a muddy makeshift grave.

I thought later that I had, at least, laid her in the earth at the foot of a mountain where ancient Korean kings and queens were buried in those sepulchers of earth like giant towering breasts of soil. I buried her in the bosom of the mountain, so that she would not spend her much too finite scrap of eternity entirely motherless. There was both tenderness and dignity in that. Isn't that what was missing?

I returned to our deserted building. My co-teachers were away on a trip. I drank several bottles of straight soju lying on my pallet on the floor in an agony of despair. One little handful of kittens opened up all the other wounds. It took so little. I had only "saved" her for one week. I could not bring her all the way back into the land of the living from the brink of death. When I shared the tale later, one of my favorite students said by way of consolation, "At least she knew love." That was all I had to cling to. And isn't that all we ever have?

Reflection

By the time I met Pia in Korea in 2010, I had already begun to name, in trauma therapy in 2008, the losses that shaped me.

To understand why Diane's death dismantled me, you have to go further back—before the kitten, before Korea, before Diane's diagnosis and my own—to 1971, to the first wound I didn't realize had broken me so completely, the mother wound.

---

1. Hemingway, Ernest. *For Whom the Bell Tolls*. Scribner, 1940.

14

— • —

The Vault That Would Not Stay Shut

Why in the World Did I Cry So Long and So Hard Over Diane?

In 2002, one year after Diane died, I went to Belgium to present a paper at a sociolinguistics conference. Diane grew up in Belgium, so I attended a Sunday service at an Assemblies of God church there, it being the denomination her parents were missionaries with. I had hoped to run into someone who had known the Smeetons, but I did not.

At the service, I wept profusely. This is not all that out of line in a Pentecostal church service, but I cried harder than normal and I met a woman there who was concerned about me. She could not understand why Diane's death would have had such a profound effect on me. She had a friend who'd died of cancer, and she didn't fall apart like I did. She wasn't being critical, just bewildered. I had no idea how to justify or communicate the depth of my pain.

Since I only have my own lived experience as a point of reference, I cannot say what I would have done if I'd had a different biography. But I bet you, too, are wondering why the death of someone who wasn't even related to me tore me to shreds. Hopefully, this chapter will answer that question.

Diane was extremely precious to me, and her death was in itself very traumatic, but it also ripped open a deeper wound I did not know I had. And that is the one which, once opened, wouldn't stop hemorrhaging for seven years (and continued to bleed for several years after that).

There were three different years before Diane died when I cried every day and wanted to die. Each time I felt I had been abandoned by a friend. I had this deep conviction that my mother didn't love me or didn't love me enough, and I got very attached to people, wanting them, as I understand it, to replace the affection I never received from her.

And when those relationships would break under the impossible burden, I would feel such agonizing abandonment that I prayed over and over for God to take my life. I felt Diane was the one person who never tired of me. She almost worshiped me.

When I left her to go to Japan (because I felt that was my calling), she felt abandoned, and so did I, even though I was the one doing the leaving. I now suspect I may have even created this circumstance to some degree because abandonment had become my script. I expected to be abandoned, and perhaps some part of me felt I had to make that expectation a reality.

One of the three years I cried for the whole year was after leaving Diane in the States and going to Japan. So, it makes sense that when Diane was dying, her ghastly physical wound, which seemed to be the mother of all wounds, also symbolized my own mother wound.

Writing a Dissertation About My Mother Along the Way

Diane died right in the middle of my graduate school experience at Georgetown, just as I was finishing my coursework. She died in the summer, and I had to get right back to work in the fall. I changed my dissertation topic from narrative retellings to blind/sighted interaction—a case study of how my mother interacts with sighted interlocutors without gaze to regulate conversation.

I cried for two weeks when I let the insulation fall away and forced myself to open my emotional eyes to the family agony of my mother's blindness. I had sworn I would not do my dissertation about my mother. But here I was. And it would take me a decade to finish.

A dissertation is not just a book you write. It is an exercise in exorcism. For most people, it requires you to turn your soul inside out, assiduously searching for demons and expelling them, and then perpetually fending them off when they come back with their friends.

Knowing this, nobody with the brains God gave a goose would write a dissertation about their mother and only a very special kind of moron would write about her blind mother's blindness. Greetings. I am that moron.

Actually, I was doing that research on the side, but at one important conference, one scholar of note raised his hand after my talk and said he thought it was the most important thing anyone was doing in our field. Damn it. In that case, it seemed to me that I had no choice but to make it my dissertation topic.

My mother and I are the only two people in the universe who are still alive who were present at my brother's death (besides the baby). My trauma from that event was tied into my dissertation, but I had no idea because I didn't even know that trauma was there. This is where my denial was still very much in place. I could not remember what it felt like before the trauma was there. I was like David Foster Wallace's fish[1] being asked how the water was and saying, "What the hell is water?"

That trauma was my water. I didn't know what not having early childhood trauma felt like. I heard someone say that in med school you learn that one way you know a patient is dying is that she feels no pain. One of the implications of that fact is that you can have a deadly wound that you do not feel and are oblivious to. It can be killing you just the same.

Dissociation Posing as Badassery

I felt a tremendous amount of pain, but I didn't understand where it was coming from. When I told the story of Brian's death, it didn't hurt. I could not associate my pain with that event. I told the story flatly, mechanically. As if it had happened to someone else.

Since this torrent of grief emerged during Diane's death, I assumed her death was the source of this "new" escalated agony. Only later did I realize that her dying had cracked open something much older, something that had been waiting for years to be grieved.

Looking back now, I understand this as a kind of dissociation, a psychological response common in early trauma. When something is too overwhelming to process, the mind protects itself by separating the emotions from the memory. You still remember what happened, but you can't feel it. Not then, anyway. The story becomes like a documentary you've seen, rather than a chapter of your own life.

If you feel I have been hard on Diane for her denial, you may roll your eyes when you observe the level of my denial about the effect of Brian's death on me. There is a scene in the sitcom *Friends* where Ross finds out his wife is gay. Everyone knew but him. I think he said something like, "Why couldn't you leave a post it on the refrigerator door, 'By the way your wife is gay?'"[2]

This is how I felt about Brian's death. After my trauma therapy, everyone would say, "We always knew that was your biggest wound." I was astounded. Why didn't someone leave a note on the refrigerator door, "By the way... Brian's death is your biggest wound."

But having been through this process, I also now know that until you are ready to deal with it, you won't hear anyone else trying to tell you. In fact, people had been trying to tell me for years. When I told them the story they would say, "Oh so you blame yourself" and I would be all, "Pish, that is ridiculous. I was a child." Deaf as a doorknob. Denial is a force of nature.

Serendipity of Healing at the Brian Crossroads

While I was at Texas A&M, very notably living in *Bryan*, Texas (coincidentally the name of my brother—and if I had made that detail up, my editor would gag and make me change it), my colleague recommended Dr. Jones[3] to me. I loved Dr. Jones, a seventy-year-old retired Navy surgeon from the Midwest with a head full of snow-white hair who had been the dean of several medical schools.

He always said he became a psychiatrist because he wanted to "help people better." I think half the English Department was seeing him, but it just so happened that he specialized in early childhood grief. Hard not to feel like there was some kind of healing fairy dust all over this situation.

From 2004 to 2008, I would go and see him only when my depression was so acute that I couldn't function and I wanted to die, but after the crisis passed, I would run away and not go see him again for a long time. He told his secretary, "If this patient calls, get her in right away because she only calls when she's in dire need."

He had a real gift for using storytelling to get his patients to come around to various realizations. What was even more special about him was his willingness to tell vulnerable stories from his own biography to this end.

As I've noted, I was in some pretty hard-core denial about the root of my problem. Looking back, it seems absurd that I didn't know. But when you grow up in silence, you mistake numbness for strength. I knew I was traumatized by Diane's death. I did not believe I was particularly traumatized over the death of my brother. After all, I had been so young. I told the story in a practiced staccato without emotion.

I guess I believed myself to be almost supernaturally too strong to be affected.

Apparently, I always mentioned, "I was supposed to have his hand" in the course of my story. Thus, everyone else thought I blamed myself for his death, but this I vigorously denied.

Eventually, while I was living there in Bryan, Texas, hiding from my shrink, I felt myself abandoned by another deep connection, and I wanted to die so badly that I took myself to Dr. Jones and submitted to trauma therapy.

It took nearly four decades for that buried grief to demand its due. But once the vault was cracked, the memories came, not as a flood at first, but as a slow, reverberating ache. In therapy, the details began to take shape, and I started to feel what I had never been allowed to feel. Before I could begin to heal, I had to return to the day everything changed. I had to tell this horrific story again and again until I got to the bottom of how my own gruesome mother wound was inflicted. Let me share that with you now.

---

1. Wallace, David Foster. *This Is Water: Some Thoughts, Delivered on a Significant Occasion, about Living a Compassionate Life.* Little, Brown, 2009.

2. It turns out I misremembered this. I fused two different scenes together in my memory, but I think my memory is funnier.

3. The name "Dr. Jones" has been substituted for the original to preserve confidentiality while honoring the truth of the encounter.

15

THE MOTHER WOUND (LAST DAY OF MY CHILDHOOD)

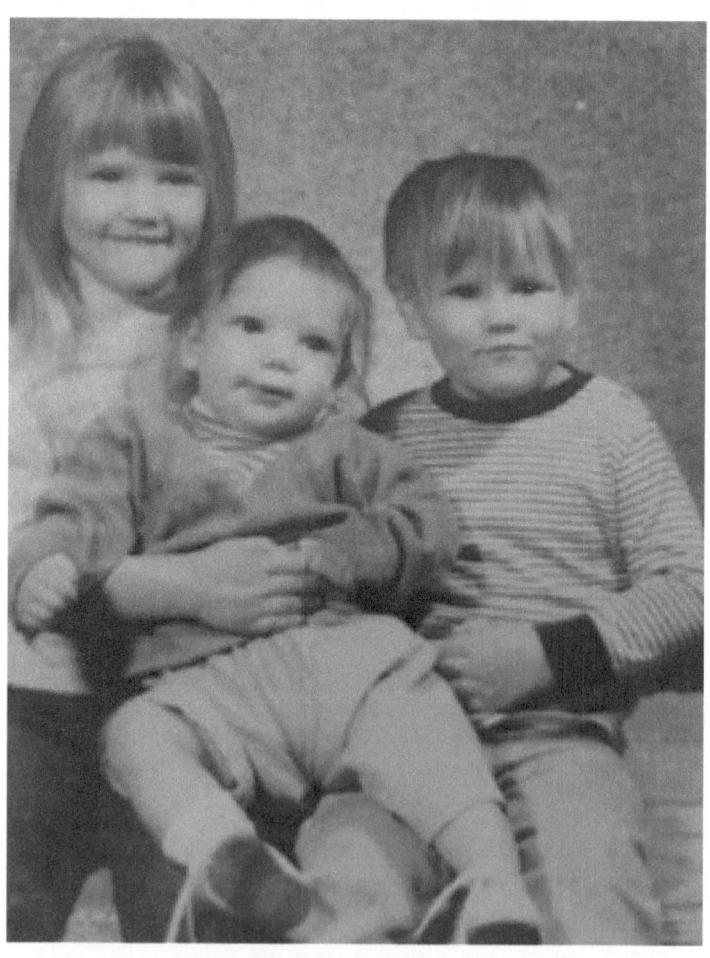

Elisa, Eric and Brian 1970

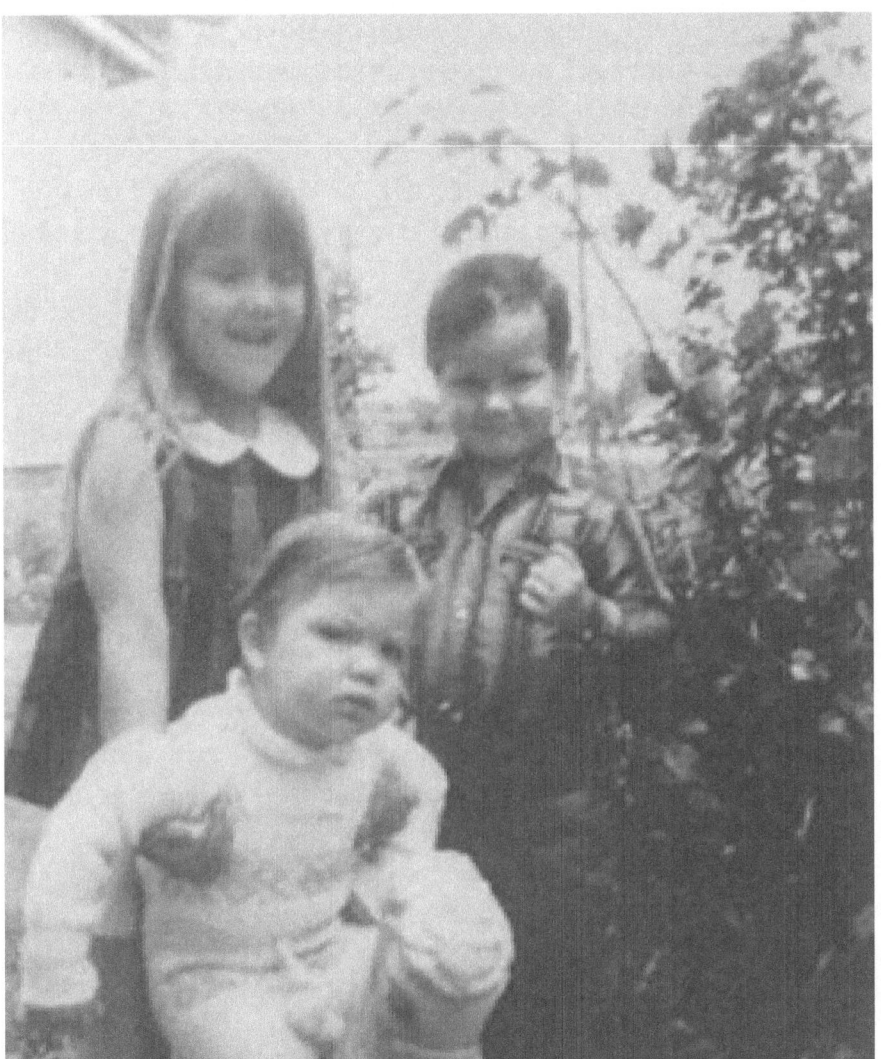

Elisa, Eric and Brian 1971

The Last Day of My Childhood

It happened on October 30, 1971. I was four and a half. Brian had just turned three. Eric was fifteen months old. Loi had not yet been born.

That year, the city decided to observe Halloween on Saturday the 30th. I say city, but really, we lived in a tiny town—Madison, Kansas. As of today, its population is 689, but there were just about 1,000 people in 1971. A single two-lane highway ran straight through town.

On one side stood my father's TV repair shop; next door was the Peter Pan Ice Cream Store. We adored the women who worked there. In hindsight, the store's name feels painfully symbolic. One of us would never grow up—but both our childhoods ended that day.

Because my mother was legally blind—she had some central tunnel vision, though even that was blurred by cataracts and color blindness—she brought along our neighbor Bonnie, who could see.

My father, weighed down by bipolar depression, couldn't get out of bed that day, so he stayed home.

As the oldest child, I was often my mother's eyes. It wasn't unusual for a child in my position to take on responsibilities far beyond her years.

Neither my mother nor I remember what our costumes were. But we kept our masks on because they were so cute. I like to imagine I was maybe a princess and Brian, maybe Superman—but that's just speculation. I'm sure he wasn't a ghost. We'd have remembered that.

I will say that our masks, whatever they were, might as well have been the faces of demons. They rendered us as blind as our mother and proved far more dangerous than anyone could have imagined.

We pulled Baby Eric behind us in a little red wagon, dressed like a bunny. That detail has stayed with me. He wasn't wearing a mask.

In his case, maybe it would have been a mercy if he had been.

I shudder to think of what he saw.

My mother, Bonnie and the baby stayed on one side of the street, and my mom sent us across the street to the ice cream store. I remember that the older ladies in the store gave us little snack-sized Snickers bars that went into our paper sacks. I was very excited about those.

When we came back out, we stood on the curb and waited for instructions.

I was forty-one years old when I woke up one Saturday in the middle of my trauma therapy and realized, "Oh my God, the truck came from the left."

I am deaf in my left ear. The problem with being deaf in one ear is not only that you don't hear things well on that side, but you cannot hear in stereo, so you can't hear direction either.

I could not see clearly because of the mask, but I also could not hear the direction of traffic. I couldn't tell whether the cars were coming or going. There couldn't have been many in a town of that size, but I clearly heard several swooshing past.

All those decades later, this detail, perhaps more than any other, helped me to accept that the accident wasn't my fault.

My mother had told us to stay put, but now she was shouting for me to come.

I hesitated because I thought I still heard a car coming.

My mother yelled again.

After some deliberation, I finally stepped out into the street and started running in blind faith.

My mother shouted, "Get your brother's hand!"

But I couldn't see my brother. I didn't even know where he was. He had been on my left on the curb, but I didn't know where he was now.

So, I did not get his hand. It wasn't a decision. She was yelling and I was running. I couldn't process the competing demand.

I kept running as fast as my little legs and my mask would allow me.

As I reached the curb on the other side, I started to feel victorious—but suddenly everyone was screaming.

Looking back, I believe that in that moment I knew that I had just ended the world, but I'm sure that's just a dramatic effect of retrospection.

The screams stretched out for eternity. Time and space and soul collapsed.

I imagine a permanent gaping hole opening up in the heart of every witness.

My little blond brother had stumbled out into the street clutching his bag of treats and walked straight under a tractor trailer. In a split second, he was dead, bathed in a small sea of blood.

I don't remember the blood. My mother told me about it.

I don't know if I didn't see it because of the mask or if Bonnie successfully shielded me from the scene when she jerked me away by the hand or if I have a mental block.

She dragged me home without speaking, without telling me what had happened.

But of course, I knew.

There could be only one reason for the screams and my brother's absence.

An Ambulance That Would Not Start

Almost forty years after the incident, I learned from my mother there was only one ambulance in town, and they were trying to mobilize it, but it wouldn't start. (Fifty years later I learned of a woman who was in the store when my mother ran in covered in blood screaming and asking for help.) The nearest hospital was twenty-five miles away.

They finally got the ambulance started. It was hot and stifling in the back and my mother felt like she was suffocating, but they wouldn't let her put the windows down because they were still working on my brother, trying to revive him. Finally, they said, "You can put the window down now." And she knew he was gone.

When she got to the hospital, she waited outside the emergency room until a doctor came out and told her in a short, clipped voice, "Mrs. Everts, your son is dead."

Meanwhile, back at the house, my grandparents and aunts and uncles began to gather. Everyone sat in stupefied silence.

I "knew" that was because, through my negligence, I had disobeyed my mother and effectively killed my brother by not getting his hand. I went around offering candy to them one by one, trying to cheer them up, but no one wanted any. They didn't look at me or talk to me.

I now understand how much agony and shock they were in. At the time, I mistook it for anger.

When I look back, it's hard not to think, "Why wasn't anybody holding that child?" But I come from one of those midwestern families where, as my uncle tells it, we show each other how much we love each other by not hitting each other hard.

We were not huggy, kissy people. And everyone was in shock. That's why no one was holding that child.

Also, I was not crying. No one was crying. We do not cry in front of anyone. If we cry, no one will ever know because no one will ever see it.

Of course, I think they may have cried in private, but I did not know that then. All I saw was the quiet unspoken horror we were all drowning in.

Perhaps if I had cried, someone would have picked me up. This occurs to me because I went to the bathroom and left the door cracked open for fear of the dark. I had some pain when I used the bathroom and made a noise, and my aunt asked me if I was ok. This seemed to be the story of my life for some time. If I had made more noise about my pain, perhaps someone would have come.

For years, I did not make any noise at all about this pain. Not even in the privacy of my own mind.

After what seemed like days but was probably about two hours, maybe three, my father finally came to the house and picked me up and carried me around. He had been to the hospital. He was silent.

We were standing in front of a window with our backs turned to everyone else. I remember how, with great foreboding, I asked him first the question I thought was safer, "How is Mom?"

He said flatly, "She's fine."

"And how is Brian?"

In the same matter-of-fact tone, "He's dead."

No mollycoddling or pussy footing around the truth. These are the facts. They don't change just because you're four.

And that was the unceremonious end to my childhood.

The Deadly Silence

I didn't just not see my parents cry that day. I never saw them cry. (I saw my mother cry in church sometimes in my teen years, but I never saw her mourn in any way I could recognize). And I don't remember ever crying about it myself (until the trauma therapy). I felt sick and horrified and lonely, but I didn't cry. As far as I knew, we did not grieve. We didn't talk about it. We stuffed.

I had recurring nightmares throughout my childhood and adult life that I was in charge of a baby who turned into a lizard or a package of Kool-Aid, or something not alive. It was always my fault. The baby died or disappeared on my watch. I would wake just as I had to give account to the parents of what I had let happen. I dreamed that as recently as last year.

I am pleased to report that I have had the dream in reverse recently, where I saved the baby. I believe that to be evidence of the healing that has taken place in the depths of my psyche.

I would eventually learn that I cried in my sleep, well into adulthood. And as I grew up, I departed from my family's affective norms and became an expressive person who cried with some frequency.

By the time Diane died, I was a gushing geyser (although I still didn't cry about Brian—at least, not knowingly). I could not connect my emotions with the accident or its aftermath.

Why Was My Mother Always Angry?

My mother was angry during a lot of my childhood. Granted, she had a lot to be angry about. Blindness, poverty, grief, my father's mental illness and unemployment.

Anger, Dr. Jones always reminded me, is a screen emotion. It's safer than expressing the pain and terror you might be feeling. Anger propelled my mother through great difficulty and helped us keep body and soul together.

As I mentioned, I was the oldest child and often functioned as my mother's little visual assistant. Of course, it was frustrating for her to have only a child helping her and I'm afraid I often messed things up. Thus, I perceived a lot of the anger to be about me and ultimately came to realize I believed she had stopped loving me when Brian died.

I believed that the moment he died, my mother stopped loving me and no one else would ever love me again either. So naturally I hated myself and every time someone abandoned me (usually because I came to cling too tightly and sometimes because my trauma was too much), it confirmed my conviction that I had rendered myself entirely unlovable.

I eventually learned that my mother never blamed me and had no idea I felt that way. (On the other hand, my father did blame me, at least at times. I remember sitting on the rail of our front porch when my dad came to visit when I was about fourteen, after the divorce, and him casually saying, "With a little sense you could have saved your brother's life.")

Nevertheless, facing this wound brought an installment of healing to me and to my relationship with my mother.

Retraumatized

While I was going through this therapy and the Pandora's box of trauma was open, however, I had two horrible experiences. The first was a devastating retraumatizing experience with a movie. It was *AI*[1] by Steven Spielberg (but it could have been by Stephen King!).

In the film, a little robot "boy" named David is adopted by a family whose biological child was in a cryogenic state due to an illness. The robot boy had a switch I think (there's no way I'm going to watch that movie again to verify!) which the parents could activate if they decided to keep him—it was a switch to activate unconditional love. They decided to activate it, and after that David loved his mother as much as any human child.

Unfortunately for David, the other child came out of his illness and returned home. Of course, he was loved, and David was now an afterthought, just excess baggage. David tried to compete with the other boy for his mother's love, and one day he and the real boy had a fight at the pool. David fell into the pool, and everyone just left him there at the bottom of the pool. At this point in the movie, I was crying pretty hard.

But it got worse. Instead of taking David back to the factory to be destroyed, the mother let him go in the woods to fend for himself. He eventually spent millennia, trapped at the bottom of the ocean, still "alive," still praying to the Blue Fairy to become real—so his mother would love him again. I cried until I almost hyperventilated. I stood over the sink and cried my guts out. No one told me it was a story of psychological horror. The scene was retraumatizing and split my mother wound wide open. It helped confirm for me that we were right on track in the trauma work. This was indeed the core of my woundedness.

If I needed any more evidence, I had a major blowout, a psychological breakdown at work during this time. There was another professor, let's call her Sarah, who was well known for her surliness. I don't remember the fine details, but she told me I should already be done with my dissertation (which was a big wound in itself; remember, my dissertation was about my mother) and I got an email saying she wanted to meet with me.

I freaked out. I started crying in the mailroom and a wonderful woman who was an administrator at the time and an ethics professor, took me in her arms and then took me in her office and let me cry.

Nevertheless, I went back to my office and cried my guts out and felt like I wanted to die. I wrote to the head of the department and told him I was so upset I just wanted to float away in the ocean. He misinterpreted this as a suicide threat and followed the suicide protocol, which involved having the campus police come and carry me away in a black and white to see a campus therapist.

Before they came, my department head realized he had made a mistake as he stayed with me in my office while I cried, but there was no way to halt the process once it had been initiated.

My own psychiatrist, Dr. Jones, could not take me that evening because he did not have access to a hospital if I needed it. But the next day was Saturday, and he saw me for at least three hours (he did not charge me and even gave me money for medicine). He said he felt like this had happened because he had pushed me too hard in therapy. We got through this, and it just became part of the trauma therapy journey.

Holey, Wholey, Holy

The accident that killed my brother was like a black hole that sucked up Brian, my mother, my childhood, and about a thousand acres of my soul.

It shattered my world and rewrote the script of my identity, from loved to unlovable, from innocent to heinously guilty, from enough to too much and not enough all at once.

But that script is no longer mine. Dr. Jones helped me rewrite it.

I have stared down the silence. I have grieved the boy, the mother, the childhood, the injured soul. I have walked back through every room of that haunted house, turned on the lights, and named what lived there.

And now, I walk forward. The hole closed and coughed up its captives. I became whole again.

The healing process, so holy.

---

1. *A.I. Artificial Intelligence*. Directed by Steven Spielberg, performances by Haley Joel Osment, Frances O'Connor, Jude Law, and William Hurt, Warner Bros., 2001.

16

— · —

FREE HAND-ME-DOWN EPIPHANIES, LIGHTLY USED

How Did We Get to the Point of Closing the Hole? (Free Epiphanies, Better Than Snacks)

I can't speak from the clinician's point of view, but I can tell you what it felt like from the inside. Healing didn't come all at once—it came in layers, like peeling an onion, or maybe like revising a very old, very painful story draft.

Essentially, I told the story of Brian's death again and again—each time peeling back a little more, remembering a little deeper. I went back into the dark, scary rooms of memory and slowly reconstructed the scene.

People have said to me, "But you were only four—you can't possibly remember."

Oh, but I do. I remember it all with aching clarity. And every time I've checked my memories with my mother, she's confirmed their accuracy.

Still, there were things I didn't know—details buried, truths half-formed, connections I hadn't yet made. It wasn't until I walked the story all the way through in therapy that the dots began to connect. That's when the shape of it changed—when the black hole began to lose its pull. With every retelling, more revelations surfaced, more pieces of the puzzle that had been buried under years of silence, shame, and misinterpretation.

The final version of the story, the one I carry now, is the one where I understand that I was not responsible for my brother's death. I understand the genesis of that incredible mother wound. And I finally know without a doubt that my mother never blamed me, that she, in fact, loves me more than life, and that many other people love me too (as it turns out, I am actually quite lovable—who knew?).

Along the way, I had a whole series of revelations that helped me come to those final conclusions. I'm going to share them with you, just in case you don't happen to have a Dr. Jones of your own at the ready.

If there are any parallels in your experience, maybe you can absorb a few of these hard-earned epiphanies vicariously—on the cheap. (You're welcome.)

Epiphany One: Diane's Death Was the Key to Brian's

One, Diane's death ripped open this mother wound and crippled me, almost fatally. It wasn't just grief—it was a full-body rupture, a soul-level unraveling. Her death didn't merely trigger sadness; it detonated something buried so deep I hadn't even known it was there.

What I thought was unbearable pain over losing Diane turned out to be the unlocking of decades of stored sorrow—abandonment, guilt, the silent ache of feeling unloved by my mother, and the primal helplessness of a child left to make sense of a broken world.

Diane's tenderness toward me had been a kind of salve, a stand-in for what I didn't receive in early childhood. So, when she died, it felt like the last person who truly saw me had vanished, and with her, all my scaffolding collapsed. I was left exposed, raw, flailing, and unprotected in the storm of grief I had outrun for decades.

This goes back to chapter one and Diana Gabaldon's quote that one grief is the key to them all. Brian's death was the key to them all.

Epiphany Two: Children Are Not Developmentally Capable of Grieving

Children are not developmentally capable of grieving, and I had not grieved my brother's death. That's not a metaphor—it's neurodevelopmental fact. At four and a half, I simply didn't have the cognitive or emotional tools to process a loss of that magnitude. My brain did what it had to do to survive: it filed the event away in some deep, locked chamber, sealed with silence and fog. For decades, I truly believed I had dealt with it. I would tell the story of Brian's death with a kind of narrative polish—detached, flat, almost proud of how little it hurt.

I mistook that numbness for strength. I honestly thought that not feeling anything made me some kind of badass, a person forged in fire and immune to pain.

But of course, that wasn't resilience—it was trauma masquerading as toughness. That false bravado kept me going for years, but it also kept me severed from my own heart.

Oh, hubris and denial—my old companions. I have mixed feelings about being rid of you. You got me through a lot, but you also kept me from healing.

It turns out, feeling nothing is not a sign of strength. It's a symptom. And eventually, the grief I had locked away came pounding on the door, demanding grief's rent.

Epiphany Three: Grieving Parents Pull Away from Surviving Children

One of the most pivotal revelations was understanding that when a parent loses a child, they often pull away emotionally from their surviving children—not because they love them any less, but because the very act of staying present becomes unbearable.

I had always interpreted my mother's distance as a kind of rejection, as evidence that I was unlovable or, worse, blamed.

But this new lens helped me reframe her behavior not as a reflection of my worth, but as a symptom of her own profound grief. She had been broken, too. Her withdrawal wasn't about me—it was about her own survival.

That insight changed everything. I had spent so many years internalizing her silence, confusing her numbness and anger with condemnation. But now I could see that it wasn't about what I had done or failed to do. Her distance wasn't personal, it was protective, even if it had wounded me deeply.

That was huge.

Epiphany Four: Mothers and Daughters Tend to Merge

Closely related to this was another profound discovery, one I've since seen echoed in the lives of many women I know. Mothers and daughters often have porous boundaries. Their identities can blur, especially in times of stress or grief, and a mother may unconsciously see her daughter not as a separate, sovereign being, but as an extension of herself.

And when a woman is hard on herself—as my mother undoubtedly was—she can become equally hard on her daughter without even realizing it.

This explained so much. My mother's criticism, her frustration, her sharpness—they weren't necessarily about me at all. They were reflections of her own internal struggle, projected onto the person who was, perhaps, in some ways most like her.

This realization didn't erase the pain, but it made room for compassion. I stopped trying to earn her love through perfection and began to understand that both of us had been trapped in roles we didn't choose, shaped by forces neither of us fully understood.

Epiphany Five: Talking about the Event Would Be a Gift to My Mother

A fifth surprise was learning that talking to my mother about this event would be a gift to her. I had spent so many years protecting her from my feelings, (and protecting myself from what I was afraid would be her indifference to my feelings), assuming she wouldn't want to revisit the pain. And I think I even feared at some level that she would actually blame me with words, on the record, in a way I could not escape.

But when I finally opened up this conversation, I discovered something unexpected—she welcomed it. It gave her a chance to share her own memories and grief, which had long been buried beneath layers of silence and stoicism.

In speaking aloud what had once been unspeakable, we created space for a kind of emotional intimacy that had rarely existed between us. For the first time, we weren't just mother and daughter—we were co-witnesses, co-survivors of something unspeakably tragic.

I think it brought healing to both of us, not only for the loss of my brother but also for the years of distance that loss had driven between us.

Epiphany Six: Trauma Therapy Isn't Remembering; It's Reliving

While I went through the therapy, it wasn't like I was remembering the trauma. I was reliving it. I wasn't in a therapist's office, at the grocery store, in my classroom—I was back in the street, back in the scream, back in the ensuing silence. I was there.

As I had done when Diane died, I physically staggered around campus like a drunk under the weight of grief. I felt like someone had their hands around my esophagus and was squeezing it tight. It was literally a choking grief. I didn't just recall what happened—I became the child who couldn't breathe, the big sister who couldn't find him to pull him out of the truck's path, who didn't even know there was a truck.

I called my mother, and we had many conversations about it. Dr. Jones was right. It was a gift not only to me but to my mother to be able to talk about it. We had no one else on earth who shared the experience to discuss it with.

I learned a number of important details that shed more light on the experience. By taking apart my fossilized childhood story and reconstructing the narrative, I was able to get my memory of the event and my emotions back together. It was like I had sealed off the grief in some chamber of my soul, and now that I was going back in, the seal broke, and fresh grief gushed out of me like it had just happened.

But this terrible pain was actually a sign of the healing. The great chasm between memory and emotion was healing, and the evidence was that I could feel again.

Epiphany Seven: A Method to the Madness (Death Anniversaries)

Because I had been seeing Dr. Jones over the course of five years, he was able to see patterns that I would not have believed had he not documented them. It turned out that my worst passively suicidal episodes and relationship blowouts coincided with the anniversaries of Diane's and Brian's deaths (the event in the English department happened around late October).

I previously did not believe there was anything special or important about specific dates, but it turned out my breakdowns were predictable. Your soul has an internal clock that keeps track.

This revelation in itself was when the penny dropped for me. It confirmed for me that Brian was the deep, unhealed wound I was suffering so much from all along. Until that time, I didn't believe it.

Soul Level Rituals of Repair

Dr. Jones told me a story about a woman (whom I like to call Mrs. Peabody, for reasons that will become evident) who could not stop throwing up and was hospitalized for it several times a year. It turns out this started when her father, whom she was very close to, died (vomiting a lot in the process).

A family member had sexually abused her, and she felt her father had known about it but had not intervened. Dr. Jones said, "I want you to go to your father's grave and talk to him, and then I want you to go to your relative's grave and talk to him." She went to her father's grave and forgave him. Then she went to the other man's grave and took off her underwear and peed on it. And she never vomited again.

So, he wanted me to go to my brother's grave and talk to him. I had written a song for Brian in high school, which I added verses to as the years passed. I drove to Kansas to see my family. One day, I drove out to the cemetery, which was in a very remote place, and I took my guitar and sat on his grave and played my song for him.

Where Have You Gone, My Friend (Brian's Song)
You were my darling
brother Brian
And when you died
I never stopped crying.[1]

You were my only playmate,
my first, my dearest friend.
We had a happy childhood
and I thought that it would never end.

Where have you gone my friend
and are you watching me?
I wonder if you know my thoughts,
I wonder, "What do you see?"

I saw you in my dreams last night
as I think you would be now.
I wondered at the meaning of
that wrinkle in your brow.

Do you know the secret joys

that make the living wise?
And are you hiding something there
behind those deep blue eyes?

Where have you gone my friend
and are you watching me?
I wonder if you know my thoughts,
I wonder, "What do you see?"

I will not forget the day
I failed to take your hand
to have you walk under the wheels
of an unsuspecting man.

Did you see the angels there
who came to bear you home?
And did you ask them how I would
survive down here alone?

Where have you gone my friend
and are you watching me?
I wonder if you know my thoughts,
I wonder, "What do you see?"

One day I will stand with you
on Jordan's other side.
And we will dance and laugh so hard,
we'll forget we'd ever cried.

And I will look into your eyes
and finally know what you can see.
And you will look back into mine
and see yourself inside of me.

Where have you gone my friend
and are you watching me?
I wonder if you know my thoughts,

I wonder, "What do you see?"

The clouds did not part, no angels appeared. I did not have chills or any kind of supernatural experience. But from that time, I gradually stopped wanting to die.

Stopping the Cycle

The first thing I did to stop the cycle of semi-annual meltdowns and relational blowouts was to start anticipating relational seam splitting around the important anniversaries and warn those close to me that if something happened, it probably had nothing to do with them and everything to do with the person whose death anniversary it was (usually Brian's).

Little by little over the course of about seven years, by anticipating and preparing for these incidents, I stopped having these meltdowns and stopped wanting to die. I think I had my last relationship rupture of this kind around October of 2014—I no longer wanted to die, but the relationship rupture was spectacular.

It continued to be the case that sometimes when I drank too much, until about 2017, I would cry about Brian as if the accident had just happened. This was a real bummer for my friends if we happened to be at a gathering. It was amazing how long it took to cry it all out even after the trauma therapy and healing. But eventually I did cry it all out and I never have episodes like that anymore.

Healing didn't come to me like a flash of lightning (I wonder if it ever does). It came more like that song did—one verse at a time over the course of years. I sang it until it lived in my body as well as my memory. I still carry Brian with me, not as a wound anymore, but as a presence. A melody. A heartbeat under my skin. And while the grief no longer chokes me, I still cry sometimes when I tell the story or think of him.

But these tears are not trauma tears. They're tears of healing. Not to sappify the experience too much, but they are little drops of love. And they remind me that I am healed—my emotions and my memory are one again. And remembering can be holy, even when it's hard.

So, if anything I've shared here resonates, please help yourself. Free hand-me-down epiphanies. Lightly used. Durable. Even better than snacks.

1. At the time, the line "I never stopped crying" seemed entirely appropriate. As I processed my grief journey, I realized I didn't actually cry for him until Diane died. Well, I cried in my sleep and that was probably for Brian, but I wasn't aware of it yet.

17

_—·—_

REFUGEE FROM A BONELESS CHICKEN RANCH RISING

There was a long stretch of time—longer than I care to admit—when I could barely tell whether I was recovering or just rotting like lettuce in the crisper (which for most of us, let's be honest, should really be called the _soggier_). I wasn't living, exactly. I was floppily not dead and not trying to die. Limp. Undone. And no, I was definitely not pulling myself up by my bootstraps. (Scoffs, as if I could find my boots).

Resurrection Takes Time

In my experience, rising from the dead is never instant. Even if a deadly cancer is cut out or killed by chemo, you don't wake up the next day ready to dive back into your pounding schedule of work and play. You have to heal. You may need physical therapy. You may need to learn a completely new way to live, to be in the world.

I pursued my emotional healing doggedly, if very feebly at times and I never gave up. I wandered in my bewilderness for three more years after the trauma therapy, still healing, still unraveling the knots that therapy had exposed.

It took me another seven years or so to go from regularly being suicidal to just being a nonfunctional blob (my friend John likes to describe me at this early stage as a refugee from a boneless chicken ranch as it seemed I rather lacked the strength to support my own head) to being, ultimately, a 9 to 10 out of 10 on the happiness scale every day.

You may think, "My God, it took ten years??" (That's a total of 18 years from Diane's death and 48 years from Brian's, but who's counting?). As I mentioned before, I've noticed that most people go to their graves without ever getting their deepest wounds healed. If I have a choice between ten to even fifty years and never, I'll take the former. However, it is my sincerest wish that by telling my story, some of you will be able to find your healing faster. Not fast, mind you, but faster than that.

From the Disorient to the Orient: Making My Way from Texas to Korea

So, my trauma therapy was from 2008 to 2009, and in the spring of 2009, my visiting lectureship at A&M was up, and I had to leave. I put all my stuff in storage and went to Kansas, where my dad, his doctors, and everyone in the family thought he was dying.

I don't want to be too egotistical, but it seemed like when I got there, he was pretty happy to see me, and he decided to not die for another couple of years. So, after a few weeks, I went to Arkansas to stay with a dear friend and her husband and three girls for about six months.

While I was there in October, I did have a rupture, but I didn't actually want to die, and I survived the episode. Unfortunately, I think it did do some damage to my relationship with that friend, who could not understand the depth of my trauma.

The Career that Grief Unmade

All this time, my career was dying. Totally appropriate, I suppose.

I had received a four-year teaching fellowship to do my doctorate at Georgetown University—one of the greatest honors and pleasures of my life. I had presented papers and workshops at seven conferences before I even started graduate school at Georgetown. I was president of the Graduate Students Linguistics Association for a year. I had presented at about twenty conferences by the time my trauma therapy started, including in France, Belgium, Italy, and later Germany.

I had published two seminal articles in humor and blind/sighted interaction. I was given the Emerging Scholar award by the International Society for Humor Studies in 2004 (ironically while grieving so heavily for Diane). I had taught at Georgetown, William & Mary, and Texas A&M.

I appeared to be going places. I was up and coming. And then, by 2009—when I was leaving A&M—I was apparently up and gone.

While I was at Texas A&M, I had made a connection with a graduate student from Korea who started hiring teachers from A&M through me to teach at a foreign language boarding school in Korea. Because I wasn't finished with my dissertation, I thought no one else would take me (I didn't even apply anywhere), so I "hired myself" and went to Korea.

I cried all the way to the airport because I did not want to go. The other teachers, whom I had hired, were young enough to be my daughters, but considered me their equal, because we were doing the same job. I was lonely and miserable most of the time.

One Korean teacher reached out to me, and we became very close. There was a rupture that October, but this time I knew it had nothing to do with my lovability, and I was really surprisingly strong about it. I went back to the States to get my own cat, Kiara, and bring her back (the incident with Pia had happened six months earlier) and that helped.

I nevertheless drank copious quantities of soju, that very strong Korean liquor. I'm not sure how my brain and liver survived.

But in the midst of all that emotional turbulence and all that alcohol, something amazing happened: I finished my dissertation. I defended it over a conference call that stretched across time zones—from Korea to Germany to the U.S. I had pulled myself through the fire, one thread at a time, and stitched together something complete.

Winding My Way Back *Home* to Northern Virginia/DC

In 2012, my two years were up at the school, and I went back to Kansas, where this time my dad was genuinely dying. He was in a very nice nursing home (thanks to my sister's involvement), and I went to see him three or four times a week and just hung out with him all day. I would have gone every day, but I didn't have a car. I often walked five miles to the facility rather than pay $40 for taxis to and from.

He had dementia related to his Parkinson's, but they gave him a dementia patch, and this seemed to also help with his bipolar disorder, so in fact, he was the healthiest and most grounded I had seen him since my childhood. To me, it felt like I had gotten my father back, and it was a tremendous gift.

When I told him about my grief journey, he was still a little far away mentally, but he said, "We have to get you some counseling!" It was quite precious. I had a very healing time with him during those months. I had come in March, and he passed away in July.

There was a rupture between my sister and me in front of his deathbed, which was epic, but it was about her wounds, not mine. I survived, though

I rather wanted to die for several months that summer while I was staying with my mother, who was very tired of me occupying her very small house. I thought this would be a swell time for her to be warm and welcoming and loving to make up for some of the past, but this did not happen.

In my own family, I felt lonelier and more abandoned than ever.

Fortuitously, my friend Karen from Georgetown — yes, the same Karen who rescued me the day my car was booted in April of 2001 — now an assistant dean at Northern Virginia Community College, came to the rescue again by calling me and telling me they had an opening starting in October.

I had no place to live and virtually no money, so I reached out to my dear friend Stacy, whom I knew from that little church plant from 2001. Stacy, God bless her, said, "This is where you belong. I will find you a place to live or die trying." And she did.

She connected me to a church friend named John who had a room in his house for rent. I called him, and we bonded over some weird religious groups we both knew of (weird religious groups being his specialty).

There just happened to be an Everts family reunion in Virginia Beach the weekend before I was to begin teaching, so my stepfather, Gail, drove me to Chicago to meet up with my Uncle Jim, who was himself like a father to me, and we drove out to Virginia together (with my beloved cat).

My Chosen Bonus Family Appears Like the Avengers, in Costume

John lived two blocks away from Mike and Tina, with whom he was great friends, and who were also from the same church Stacy had been a part of. On Halloween, they had a big party, and John took me over there to meet them. Tina was wearing a couch. I mean she had taken the vinyl off of a couch and fashioned it into a primitive outfit which she was wearing as Tarzan's wife or something.

She was also a beader and took me down in the basement to see her jewelry stuff, and we bonded instantly.

The next day John called me and asked me if I was free. Tina had fallen down in the parking lot at work, writhing in pain with twisted intestines, the ambulance came and took her to the hospital, and her 96-year-old grandfather, who was visiting, had no one to be with him. So of course, I said I'd go hang out with Grandpa (who was a total delight).

Their friends (soon to be mine) Ken and Maranda came to the house, and we all went to the hospital together and hung out. Various friends from the aforementioned church came by to bring food and company. They were supposed to have another party which couldn't happen because Tina was in the hospital having surgery, so they brought the party to her.

Dee and her family came in costume. Dee was Margo Rita in a cute skirt with a sparkly green mask and high white vinyl boots carrying a pitcher of "lemonade" which was, of course, really the most delicious margaritas, which we had in the hospital, and it was awesome. I knew we were destined to be great friends.

These people were all very close to Stacy, and they just took me in as part of their family. One of our group members was basically a tree surgeon, which was appropriate because it was just as if I had been grafted into this healing tree of beautiful people (and this time there were no amputations). It was a match made in heaven. So that October there were no ruptures, only bonding and joy. I was welcomed into a family of friends who loved me unconditionally for exactly who I am. Stacy was right; this is where I belong.

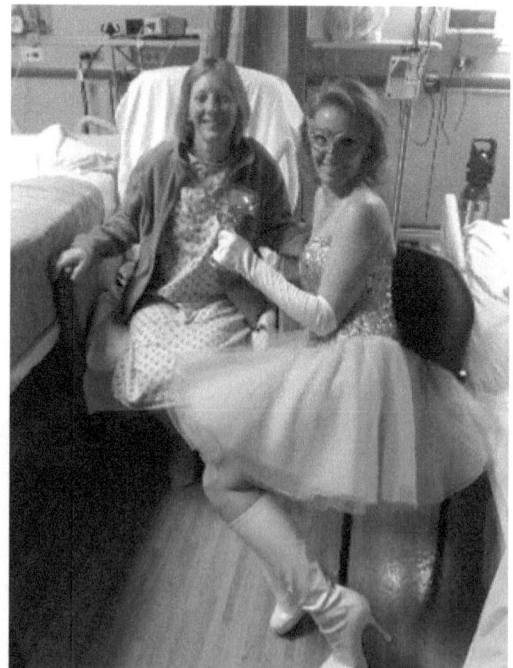

Tina in the hospital with Dee as Margo Rita

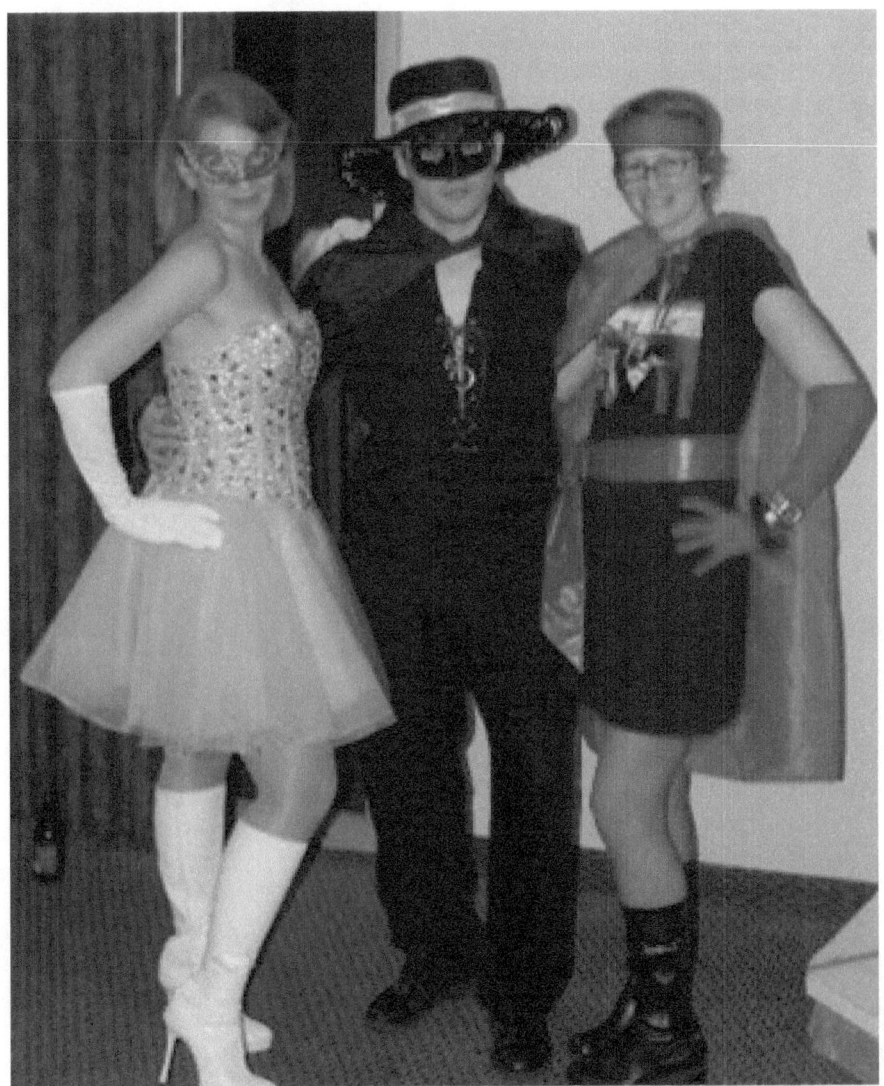

Dee, Ken, and Maranda

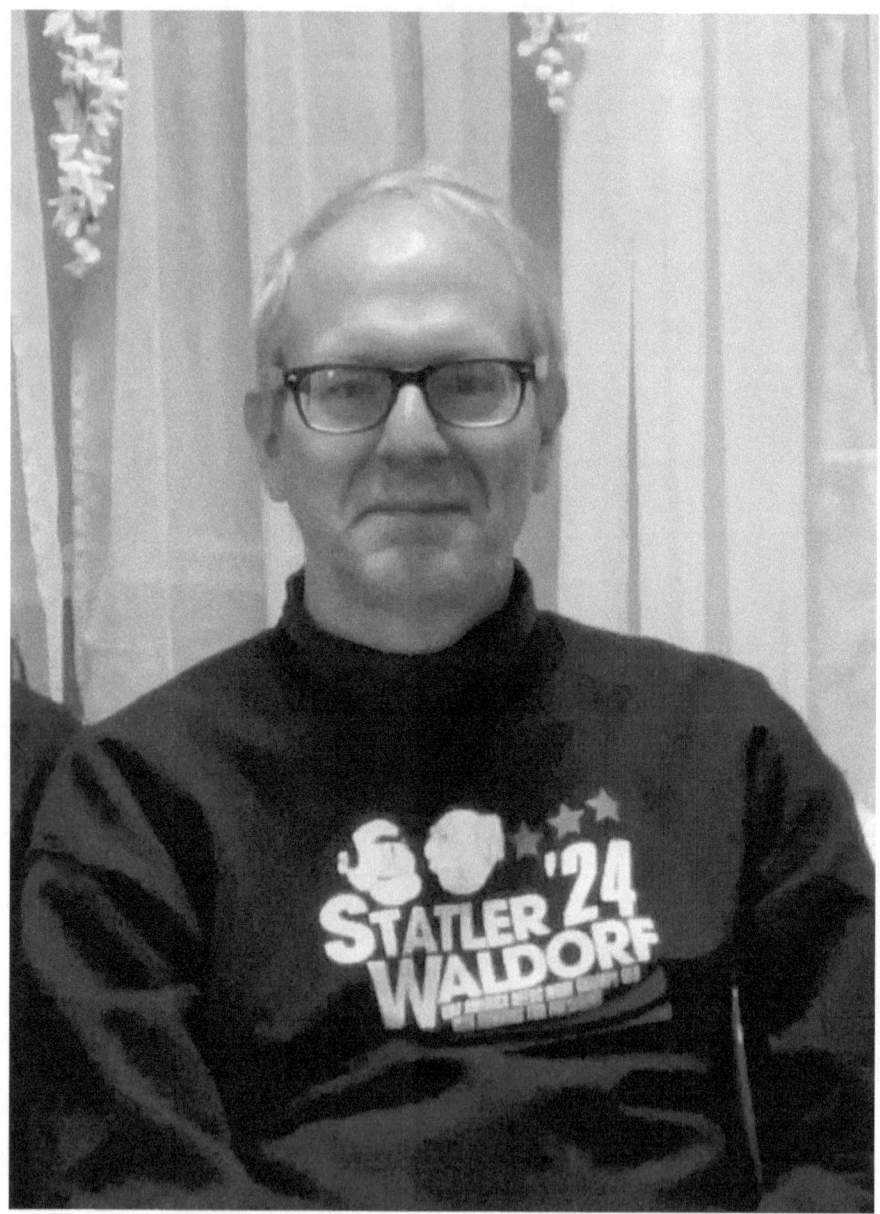

John

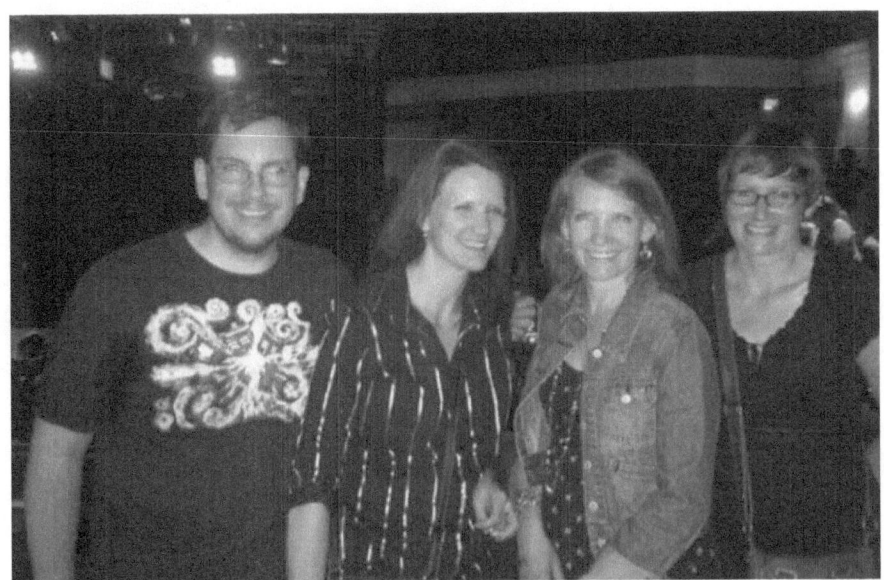

Mike, Elisa, Dee, and Maranda at a Concert 2013

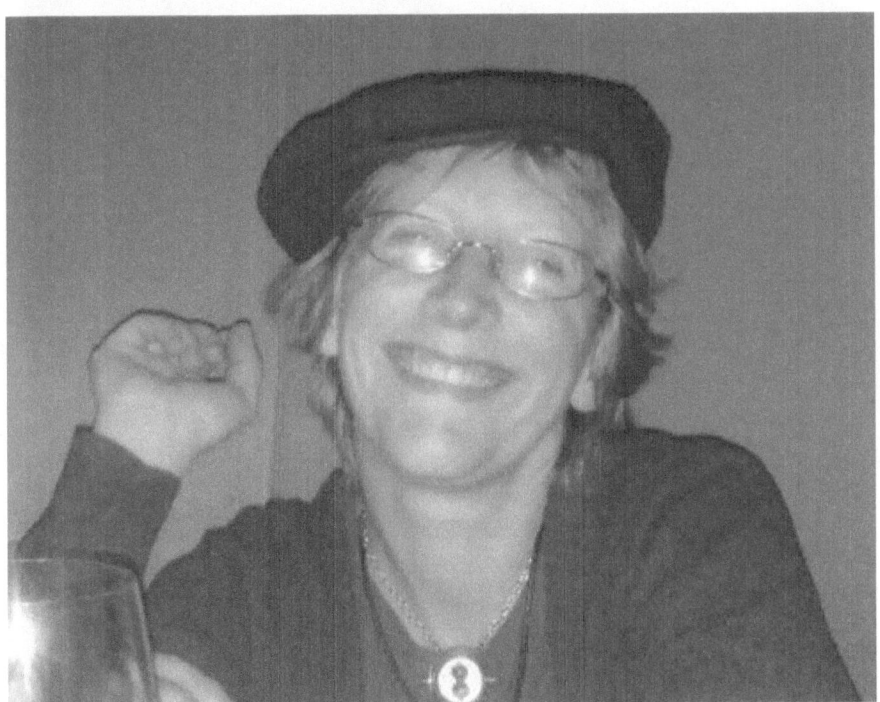

Tina at the Winchester

There was a Bar Louie restaurant down the street, which we all used to frequent together, calling it *The Winchester*, after a tavern in *Shaun of the Dead* where everyone went to hide out during the zombie apocalypse. Wonderful times were had at *The Winchester*, especially on Tuesday five-dollar burger nights.

This was the most alive I had been in years, though since I was an uber introvert and still very much an underemployed blob, I still hid in my room "caving" for days at a time. It was a big deal to get me out to burger night. John was great at dragging me out into social events.

I was an adjunct ESL (English as a Second Language) teacher at NOVA, needless to say a job I could have done without a PhD in linguistics, but it did help. I was happy at my job. I was always of the mind that teaching of any kind, but particularly ESL teaching, is a beautiful way of loving people.

I didn't have a car, and I had to walk a mile to the bus stop, take two buses, two trains and a shuttle just to get from Herndon to my job in Annandale. In some ways my life was still a suckfest.

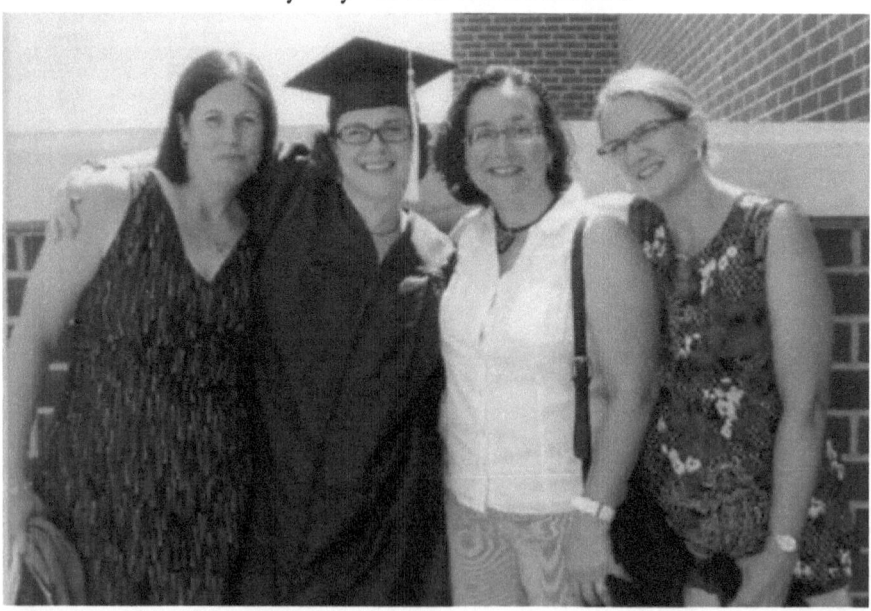

Julie, Erin, Lena, and Me

Lena's House of Becoming

I had, since Diane died, a terrible fear of talking on the phone, listening to and answering phone messages, and opening and replying to emails and snail mail. (A psychiatrist at NIH would later explain to me that this was consistent with complex PTSD.) As a result of this disability, I missed an email about what classes I wanted the next semester, and as a result, I was not given any. With no car and no income, I didn't know what to do.

So, I asked my friend Lena, who lived in Pennsylvania, if I could come live with her for a while and cook and garden and help with remodeling her house in exchange for room and board. This turned out to be a wonderful experience that I would liken to rehab. There was another woman living there, going to grad school, and also benefitting from Lena's magnanimity. It was kind of Lena's House of Becoming.

Lena might be the most positive human being I have ever met. She is a great fan of Wayne Dyer, Tony Robbins, Les Brown, Zig Ziglar, and Rhonda Byrne, among others in that arena. We read and listened to their books constantly and focused on gratitude, goals, and transforming negative thoughts into positive ones.

I developed a spiritual practice I faithfully did every morning. I wrote a long manifesto, which I read aloud and recorded and listened to often. I wrote and practiced mantras. I put together a wonderfully imaginative vision board, so much of which has already come to fruition.

I don't think these practices depend on a mystical law of attraction to work. They are focusing devices, and when you focus the mind, you can achieve great results. This applied to such things as my goal to lose 20 lbs (I lost 50 by 2020) and to read many books.

I had always considered myself a reader, but outside of school, I don't think I read more than ten books a year. But I read almost 100 in 2015 after making a goal to read 75. Last year I read 180. That practice alone has been truly transformative.

However, I can't explain how two of the biggest things on my board came to be. One was a car, and the other was a job in DC. My uncle came to visit, and we went to another family reunion together. On the way back, he announced out of the blue that he was buying me a car.

Shortly thereafter, I got an email from my friend John, who had a job for me at a small private university. The timing was amazing. I couldn't have done the job without the car, and I didn't ask for either one. The job started out as ESL instructor and in two months I became Director of ESL, and shortly after that, I became an associate dean.

Never Too Late

My friend Dee (aka Margo Rita) had given me the book StrengthsFinder[1] for my birthday during this time, and by doing its assessment I was reminded how much I love writing and public speaking. I also knew I needed to be in community. So, I started going to Toastmasters, which was a real game changer in many ways.

As an introvert, the first weeks of visiting were brutal, but I finally made friends and got really involved. It had me writing for my speeches, speaking, and making so many friends. I joined several clubs, and I was out of the house multiple times a week. I'm sure all my bonus family friends were like, "Who are you and what have you done with Elisa?"

This reminds me that Dee also gave me a birthday card with a quote attributed to George Eliot, "It's never too late to be what you might have been,"[2] which I posted on the wall near my bed, and which was a source of great inspiration.

Another goal I made was to join a church, which I did in 2017. I became very involved and soon became a lector. This gave me the opportunity to do a little public speaking and also to minister to people's souls, which has always been a calling of mine.

In the beginning, I was so nervous my hands shook, but over time I got very comfortable behind the lectern. I made many wonderful friends there and got involved in the church's ministry to provide meals for people without stable housing, as well.

That year I was given the "Spirit Award" at church for my contributions to the church community. All of these things made me come alive. They were all part of this beautiful resurrection of my life.

The college I was working at closed in December of 2017, and I was unemployed for eight months. During that time, I stayed involved in Toastmasters and church, and I wrote about 100 poems. 18 of them got published (some poems, some creative nonfiction). I had a couple of blogs that kept me creative and getting wonderful feedback on that creativity.

This time unemployment did not unravel my identity. I stayed grounded in all my spiritual practices. In the fall of 2017, I got a job teaching at NOVA again, at a different campus.

In 2019, I was the District 29 International Speech[3] champion after winning the club, area, division, and finally district level speaking contests. The Toastmasters community made me feel like a minor celebrity and this was wonderful for my sense of purpose and identity.

I gave that same speech at the DC chapter of the National Speakers Association in December of 2019 and received a standing ovation. By spring of 2020, I had lost 50 pounds, I was tan and looking the best I had looked in years. I felt amazing. I was moving towards becoming a writer and public speaker.

I got a second adjunct job teaching at another university, and teaching also makes me feel purposeful and alive. Life was absolutely beautiful.

Hard Won Resurrection

I want to take a moment to point out that I still did not have a lot of money, I did not have a prestigious job, and I did not have a romantic partner, all things which many people think their happiness must be predicated upon. And yet I was a 9 or 10 out of 10 on a happiness scale of 1 to 10 every day. My resurrection was complete. My happiness did not depend on money, professional success, or a romantic relationship.

I no longer feel like a refugee from a boneless chicken ranch. I have gone from blob to blossom (I know, eloquence is my middle name). These days, I can hold my own head high—spine and soul intact. Resurrection didn't simply restore to me the years that the locusts had eaten (to borrow a metaphor from the Old Testament). My eventual happiness didn't come from snapping back to the person I was before Diane died—it came from slowly becoming someone new.

It was born of a relentless commitment to inner work and ultimately the surrender of the identity that grief had unraveled. It took chosen family to remind me I was lovable, spiritual practice to anchor me, and creativity to light me up like a fire.

I didn't just survive by the skin of my teeth. I completely rebuilt my world from the rubble of my war-torn life. Resurrection wasn't quick or glamorous. Sometimes I felt like I had simply fallen into a bottomless hole.

But at some point, I realized I could reframe this. What if I wasn't lost in a cavernous hole? What if I was gestating in the womb of the earth? That may not be glamorous, but it is in its way very beautiful. That's what my resurrection looked like.

1. Rath, Tom. *StrengthsFinder 2.0*. Gallup Press, 2007.

2. Actually from Procter, Adelaide Anne. *"A Legend of Provence." All the Year Round*, edited by Charles Dickens, vol. 7, no. 13, 13 Dec. 1859, p. 21.

3. International Speech is just the name of the category. It doesn't mean I won the world championship.

18

—·—

RETELLING, REFRAMING, REWIRING

This is the story of how I learned to speak beauty into the broken parts of my life. The repeated telling of my hardest story, the careful reframing of its meaning, and the deliberate rewiring of my mind became the scaffolding of my resurrection. This wasn't a quick fix—it was soul work. But it changed everything.

The Real Kicker

How much do you want to kick someone when you've suffered a loss and they say something like, *Maybe it's for the best. Everything happens for a reason. It's part of God's plan?* Having come from a long line of violent women, that impulse is pretty strong for me (oh, laugh already).

The real kicker (aside from me) is that I'll be damned if suffering is not our main source of growth. We talk about Post Traumatic Stress, but not nearly enough about its sister, Post Traumatic Growth, which can be just as powerful.

I am not going to say that my journey through hell with Brian or with Diane was *good*, and I am certainly not going to say that there was some kind of divine intention behind that (which would make God a sadist), but I *am* going to acknowledge that great good can come out of great evil.

The things from which I have suffered the most are also the things through which I have grown the most. Granted, this is hard to swallow on the way into a dark night of the soul (or while you are in the middle of it).

What I *am* going to tell you is that when you retell your story—consciously and courageously—you begin to rewire your brain. The neural pathways that were once a superhighway to pain, shame, and helplessness can be remapped. Retelling is not just remembering; it is re-membering—gathering the scattered parts of yourself and reintegrating them into a new, whole self.

The Wound I Fell into Became a Door

Harvard social psychologist Ellen Langer observes, citing Epictetus, "Events don't cause stress. What causes stress are the views you take of events."[1] Storytelling is how we encode and express our view of events. A story is not just a series of events, it is the way we select and interpret them. Two different people (or the same person!) could tell several very different stories based on the same events. Trial lawyers and politicians do it all the time; it's almost a competitive sport. Largely what makes something a story is adding causes and motivations to the actions and events.I knew all of this intellectually. My PhD in Interactional Sociolinguistics focused on narrative. I knew from my own academic specialty that I needed to tell myself a different story, and I constantly urged myself to do so, but I was stuck. I just couldn't see it.

I had fallen into Diane's wound like Alice falling into some ghastly wonderland, but as I had walked willingly through that wound by staying with her all the way to the end, I walked willingly through my own wound, and it eventually turned into a doorway to healing. It was a long dark tunnel, but I found light at the end.

Until such time, I felt that I had fallen into a hole and been swallowed in my entirety. When I tried to tell people what I'd been doing since Georgetown, I'd recount my path from there to William and Mary to Texas A&M and then I'd just say, "And then I fell in a hole."

That was my narrative. I saw myself helplessly lost in a black hole. And as long as I kept telling myself that story about falling into a hole, I flailed and floundered there in that darkness. It was like quicksand. The more I struggled, the further in I sank. The more I told myself that story, the more its words wrapped around me like strangling tendrils of a powerful, malevolent octopus.

So, I fought it. Weakly at first, but eventually I picked up steam. About seven years ago, I wrote a poem I didn't fully understand until now. It captured my slow climb from grief into joy, even before I knew I was healing.

The Magical Sands of Time

July 31, 2020

Hello, Beautiful Souls. My life has been a mountain range of high peaks and deep, sometimes gorge-like valleys. About twenty years ago was one of my greatest peaks, which was soon interrupted by the trauma of losing my beloved Diane, which then triggered other, even deeper traumas), and my life began to slide swiftly down to what I hope was my deepest abyss.

Ten years ago, I was near rock bottom. Today I think I am happier than I have ever been—cancer notwithstanding.

The Magical Sands of Time

You do everything well they opined,
then it all went to hell with the wine.
And my castle washed out to the sea,
my dreams either lost or set free.
She said, "You never can tell the reason or rhyme,
for the heaven and hell in each season of time,
when you've been raptured, not swept out to sea,
when you've been captured to set yourself free."

And then I slipped under the wire,
sucked in by the ravenous deep,
stripped of encumbering desire
and secrets too toxic to keep.

Sirens wailing, arms flailing, charms failing,
to such depths I fell,
through the wishing well,
through all death, and all hell
hurtling straight to the basement floor.

But when my heart would explode,
She stepped in to reload,
and the floor gave way to a door.

Then an angel appeared
with a flower for a face

And said it was time to move on.
Not a moment to fear,
not an hour to erase,
She said it was time to move on—

Through the lands and the hands
and the magical sands of time
Through the teeming, scheming,
plot redeeming magical sands of time.

Have you not read, have you not heard?
It's all at the end of the book, you know.

Through the treasure-troving,
four leaf-cloving, fate betrothing
magical sands of time,
the nursery rhymes and the heart's crimes,
the anniversary of time and the Bard's rhymes,
all entwined in the soul's climb.

It's all at the end of the book, you know.

All the days ordained for you,
and all the doorposts stained for you,
the gifts as yet unclaimed by you—

It's all at the end of the book,
indelibly stamped on its pages,
the ineffable path of the ages.

It's all at the end

of the book,

you know.

And then one day after I wrote that poem, I was writing a speech for Toastmasters and as I reflected on the course of my life, I had this epiphany that I had poetic license over the governing metaphor of my life, and I could turn that hole inside out and make it into a mountain! I had already been rewriting all the scripts in my brain, but now I really began to tell myself a story of redemption and triumph. By 2019, I was really happy.

The Psychotherapeutic Process in an Almond Sized Nutshell

This reframing and retelling parallels the process of psychotherapy. You tell the story of your life over and over, the therapist asks provocative questions that make you reconsider your assumptions about how and why certain things happened, and the therapist knows you're getting better when you start telling your story in such a way, for instance, that you are not the victim anymore.

You are not just a person stuff happened to. You are a person with agency, able to make choices and initiate change. When you reframe your story and then retell it in a new light, you also gradually rewire your brain to think in new ways. That, in a nutshell, is how I rebuilt my life from ground zero before I got cancer.

When you reframe the past, you also reframe the present—and you can reframe the future. Your identity is largely comprised of the stories you tell about yourself; both the ones you tell others and the ones you tell yourself. When you change your story, you change who you are.

The Tonic Nectar in the Bitter Sting

A philosophically inclined baby, staring down the birth canal, might muse, *Nothing good could come from squeezing myself through that tunnel.* But not making that journey would be unthinkable. Not only is there life on the other side—there is meaning in the struggle itself.

Ryan Holiday captures this in the title of his book: *The Obstacle Is the Way,*[2] reframing adversity as opportunity. Elizabeth Gilbert echoes this, "Frustration is not an interruption of your process; frustration is the process."[3] She was speaking of art, not grief—but the parallel holds.

Paradoxically, the trauma of Diane's death led me to complete healing. I often compare it to chemotherapy: it nearly kills you to save your life. That's what her death did to me. It nearly killed me—and then it saved me. It drove me to trauma therapy. And after enduring trauma therapy, I eventually stopped wanting to die.

Healing Hidden in the Great Wound

The key to my healing, my spiritual cure, was hidden in the Great Wound. That fountain of tears, which once felt infinite, was actually drawing me back to (in Rumi's words) *the source of the source of my spring.*[4]

The wound from Diane's death cracked open the wounds of early childhood and brought them into the light, where they could finally be treated. Ultimately, I found healing and an almost inconceivable happiness. But first, I had to walk by faith through the door of that ghastly wound.

Of course, the wound I had to walk through was not Diane's—it was the mother wound of Brian's death and my conviction that on that day in 1971 I disobeyed my mother by not taking my brother's hand and thus essentially killed him. Therefore, my mother stopped loving me and would never love me again. In fact, no one would ever love me again.

That wound made me feel like I deserved all the pain in my life. That was what kept me from reaching out more to get help.

Chinese Old McDonald

Have you ever heard the Chinese Taoist "Maybe" story? It's about a farmer who experiences a series of (un?)fortunate events. First, the family horse runs away, and everybody says, "That's terrible," but the farmer is more circumspect, and he says, "Maybe so, maybe not."

After a while, the horse comes back and brings a bunch of other horses with him. The neighbors exclaim, "That's great!" The wise farmer says, "Maybe so, maybe not."

Later, the farmer's son breaks his leg when one of the new horses throws him, and of course, everyone says, "That's horrible!" The wise farmer says, "Maybe so, maybe not."

Not long after that, military recruiters come marching through the area, but because the son's leg is broken, he doesn't get drafted. Everybody in the peanut gallery says, "That's wonderful." Chinese Old MacDonald says, "Maybe so, maybe not."

Of course, the story, like our lives, could go on indefinitely. And of course, that is the point of the story. Everything is so very indefinite, so impermanent, so open for interpretation. Shakespeare sums up the basic idea rather pithily in Hamlet with, "Nothing is good or bad, but thinking makes it so." The fact that it's open for interpretation means that you get to choose the interpretation. You get to frame circumstances as you will.

No Ginger

Both the Chinese parable and Shakespeare's pith are too passive for my American tastes. They make me think of a Japanese expression, *shoganai*—"nothing can be done about it"—a phrase that always made me break out in hives. I was raised by a man who intoned throughout my childhood, "If the system doesn't work, fix the system," so surrendering to the status quo made me nuts.

Of course, *shoga* also means "ginger," and *shoganai* can mean *we are out of ginger,* so my protest was always, "Shoga aru, yo! Reizouko ni aru!"—"We do have ginger, damn it. It's in the refrigerator." My pained little pun was my way of saying: there is always something you can do.

Moving Beyond Ambiguity to Agency and Advantage

The passive view of Shakespeare's quote would be that you can see anything as good or bad as you choose. That's good (please don't say, *Maybe so, maybe not!*). It's true; you can reframe any story or situation in positive ways (or negative, if you're one of *those* people).

This is the starting point. It can get you to gratitude and from gratitude to joy and contentment. But by availing yourself of your agency in making choices and taking action, you can go even further and use your ability to reframe situations to build a present and future you choose.

Lindsey Roy, who lost one and a half legs in a boating accident, gives an insightful TEDTalk about trauma and the brain titled *Phantom Life: What Trauma Taught Me about Happiness,*[5] in which she talks about finding the "hidden advantages" in painful, traumatic situations.

Even tiny things can shift your mindset, such as observing that it is way easier to paint your toenails when you can take your foot off and put it on the table. Time-saving boon that this is, it rather pales in comparison to the hidden advantage of the beautiful compassion that her suffering evoked in her toddlers.

Her two-year-old daughter came down one day with something wrapped around her leg announcing that it was *her* prosthetic leg. And her little boy would come to cuddle with her in bed and comfort her with every stuffed animal that he owned. Those children, like the children in my sister's daycare who had my blind mother as one of their caregivers, will grow up with a level of empathy and compassion that other children do not have. They will not *other* and patronize, stigmatize and marginalize those who are different, and that is one very beautiful hidden advantage.

Mindlessness as Path to Mindfulness

Dr. Heidi Hamilton, my dissertation mentor at Georgetown, is one of the most positive and compassionate people I know. In her book *Glimmers,* based on years of conversations with a woman she called Elsie in the late stages of Alzheimer's, she finds beauty even in speech that makes no logical sense. One day, Elsie was narrating the act of cleaning her glasses—every motion, every thought—and Heidi realized: there was no "information" here, only connection.

She said, "Whenever we talked, we were talking 'just to talk.' And to experience the peace that enters the soul when two people take the time to sit and enjoy whatever comes their way."

As Alzheimer's erases past and future, it anchors both patient and companion in the present. That enforced here-and-now can be a rare gift. Mindlessness, paradoxically, can lead to mindfulness—a reframing that has stayed with me.

Re: Retelling, Reframing, and Rewiring

In even the most horrible circumstances, losing one's body, losing one's mind, losing one's life, there are still these glimmers of positivity and light about us to be savored. Finding these and savoring them is a way to keep the darkness from entirely swallowing all our light.

Sometimes our situations are equal parts joy and suffering, but we obsess about the suffering and neglect to appreciate the substantial joys that are also present. Retelling, refocusing, and reframing are critical to rewiring your mind to the end of resurrection. Seeing the joy that is already present is the door to ushering in more joy.

DIY Resurrection

The point is happiness is not nearly as dependent on circumstances as we tend to believe. It's not completely dependent on things that are outside of our control. There are two reasons for this. One, we can reframe our circumstances in positive and life-giving ways and two, we can make choices that change or affect our circumstances.

There are so many choices we can make, no matter what our circumstances are. And it is those choices that are within our control that can transform our lives. As I wrote this book and retold my story for you, I went back and reviewed the choices that I made that transformed my life.

I found ten tools that I used to resurrect my life. Ten choices that have made all the difference for me. And those tools are the focus of the next chapter.

---

1. Langer, Ellen J. *Counterclockwise: Mindful Health and the Power of Possibility.* Ballantine Books, 2009.

2. Holiday, Ryan. *The Obstacle Is the Way: The Timeless Art of Turning Trials into Triumph.* Portfolio, 2014.

3. Gilbert, Elizabeth. *Big Magic: Creative Living Beyond Fear.* Riverhead Books, 2015.

4. Moezzi, Melody. *The Rumi Prescription: How an Ancient Mystic Poet Changed My Modern Manic Life.* TarcherPerigee, 2020.

5. Roy, Lindsey. *"What Trauma Taught Me about Happiness."* TEDxKC, 2017, https://www.youtube.com/watch?v=IUw8z7laPuI .

DIY RESURRECTION: THE TOOLS I USED TO RECLAIM MY LIFE

I wish I could tell you that when I found myself in hell I sat down and mapped out a clear strategy for getting out of there post haste and then did so with a hop, skip, and a jump. In fact, I did not approach my resurrection with a clear strategy.

I didn't have a map or a guide. I bumbled along and figured it out as I went. I did a lot of things that didn't work before I found the things that did. But once I made it through the gauntlet and reached this beautiful place of happiness, I went back to examine my story and identify the tools I used in my makeshift DIY resurrection tool kit.

In this chapter I'm first going to mention some of the things I tried that didn't work. I'm then going to identify ten specific tools that I now realize made all the difference. These are not tools you have to go to Home Depot for. They are mostly tools you already have in your kitchen drawer.

What Didn't Work (In Case You Were Wondering)

I think you can see these failed efforts pretty clearly in the story I have told you, but if I try to summarize what didn't work I think there are four main strategies (I'm calling them strategies, though there was nothing strategic about them) that were absolute duds.

First, I guess I unconsciously believed that time alone would heal my wounds—as if healing were on some kind of cosmic timer. If I could just hang on long enough, surely the pain would fade, and healing would begin.

But in reality, I almost got gangrene. Not literally (though I did wear the same yoga pants for a concerning number of days), but emotionally—I let the wound fester. Time didn't heal anything I wasn't also willing to face. It's also probably worth noting that until I had therapy, I unconsciously believed that I deserved to suffer because I was guilty of my brother's death so that dragged out the fruitless waiting even more.

Second, I tried to stay busy. This is a classic tactic—just keep moving and maybe you can shake the grief off. This worked great when I was in the swirl of activity with classes and students and most people did not even know that I was falling apart in private. But my academic job didn't support the busy tactic very well. I taught fifteen hours a week and had tons of holidays. That left me plenty of time to fall apart in slow motion.

Which led to my third strategy: hiding. Many psychologists call it "caving." I called it Tuesday. I could spend entire weeks in my house without stepping outside. I told myself I was introverting. Really, I was avoiding—avoiding people, avoiding the terrifying vulnerability of being seen in pain. But keeping people out didn't protect me. It just prolonged the pain.

And finally, I kept trying to claw my way back to who I had been *before*. I believed that if I could just find the old trail, I could get back on it and carry on. But the old me died with Diane. That version of me—passionate about research, focused, pre-grief—was gone. I had to stop chasing the ghost of Elisa Past and start reaching for the Elisa I was becoming. I had to accept that I wasn't going *back*. Healing meant choosing forward.

And forward meant letting my soul take the lead. I still love academia. I love watching lightbulbs go off in students' minds. But I get goosebumps when their hearts crack open. One of the most meaningful things a student ever told me was this: "I've learned more about love in your linguistics class than I ever did on a Sunday morning." That one line told me I was on the right path—not the old path, but the one emerging under my feet as I walked.

Still, it took me several years to fully trust it. I kept looking back, wondering if I should return to who I used to be. But eventually, I stopped trying to reroute the journey and started walking with intention. That's when the path began to rise up to meet me.

So, that's the short list of what didn't work—strategies that left me lonelier, more exhausted, or more buried in the dark gulf of grief. But eventually, I started trying new things. Not all at once, not with a grand plan, and definitely not with a blueprint or even a Pinterest board. Just little shifts. Small, scrappy, soul-saving moves.

In this chapter, I'm going to share ten tools that, in hindsight, made all the difference. Once I had named the ten tools that truly helped me heal, I went back and checked the research, and sure enough, there's solid science behind each of them as powerful contributors to happiness and well-being. I've tried to provide you with at least one research anchor for each tool.

You don't need a trip to Home Depot or a personal transformation retreat in Bali. These are everyday tools, most of them are already in your kitchen drawer or tucked in your junk basket by the fridge. You've probably used most of them before, just perhaps not with great intentionality. But used with intention, they can poke a hole in that canopy of darkness I mentioned in my introduction and let in the light.

The Tools in My Personal DIY Resurrection Kit

Just like that kitchen drawer you open without thinking, the one full of rubber bands, pens, Chinese takeout menus and half-dead batteries, you're probably so used to the tools inside you that you don't even notice them anymore. But they're in there.

The only item in my toolbox you might not already have is a trauma-informed therapist, but even that one is findable, and well worth the search. A trip to Home Depot will not kill you. On the contrary, it could save your life.

1 Found a Trauma Therapist, Psychiatric Care

The beginning of my resurrection was healing from trauma. Unfortunately, it took three or four years after Diane died—and nearly forty years after Brian died—for me to find the right kind of help. I sincerely hope you won't have to wait as long.

If trauma is part of your story, I urge you: find a therapist who is trained in trauma work. You must get your wounds treated before you can begin to heal, and you must heal before you can truly flourish. You may also need medication. Medication itself will not fix you, but it can help stabilize the chemical chaos in your brain long enough for therapy to start working. In my case, there is real mental illness in my genetics. My father suffered from bipolar disorder. I am fortunate never to have been hospitalized, but my father and, I am told, at least one other family member on his side have been. I can't imagine how wonderfully different my life would have been had I had good psychiatric care from childhood (and my father, too! God bless him).

As it was, I started taking antidepressants around 2003 and other medication for another diagnosis around 2015. They helped me not get sucked under by the tide of depression and swept out to sea; however, they didn't heal me or bring me happiness by themselves. They made it possible for me to focus on rewiring my brain, which was where the real resurrection power lay.

For me, the bulk of my healing came through telling and retelling my story. But make no mistake, retelling the trauma was traumatic in itself. I needed a skilled, steady therapist beside me, someone to bear witness and help me stay tethered to safety as I walked back into the fire.

At one point, the pain became so overwhelming that I nearly required hospitalization. Fortunately, I had a compassionate psychiatrist who could help me assess the level of care I needed—and remind me that even in that moment, I was not alone. For me, psychiatric care, including medication and trauma therapy, were the foundation of the house of happiness I was building.

2 Established Community

Second, I found my people—likeminded souls who love me unconditionally, just as I am. It may seem like they fell out of a tree, but in truth, every one of them came into my life because I went looking. I sought out a new church plant in 1999 (which I learned about through Diane) and that is where I met my wonderful friend, Stacy.

Stacy and I shared values that her friends also shared (spirituality, generosity, social justice, grace, intellectual curiosity, etc.). And thus, through Stacy, I inherited a whole bonus family of friends. I kept seeking. I went to Toastmasters. I joined another church. I did the research. I chased them down. And they became more than community—many of them became my chosen bonus family.

As Robert Waldinger and Marc Schulz explain in *The Good Life*,[1] decades of Harvard research reveal that the single most powerful predictor of long-term happiness isn't wealth or success, it's the strength of our relationships.

3 Developed a Spiritual Practice

I developed a prayer model based on the acronym CONNECT (Cleansing/Forgiveness, Openness, Needs of my own, Nourishment for my soul, Exaltation and Exultation, Compassion for others, and Thanksgiving/Gratitude). I spend a few minutes on each of these prayer modules every morning, usually as soon as I open my eyes and lasting from 15 minutes to an hour.

I use the Insight Timer on my phone and have a different melody/sound set for each module that helps shift me into that frame of mind. The openness module is the most like meditation. This whole practice grounds me spiritually.

Psychologist Sonja Lyubomirsky, in *The How of Happiness*,[2] points out that spiritual practices like prayer, meditation, or quiet reflection can actually help us feel more grounded, more grateful, and more alive.

4 Rewrote My Inner Narrative

The next element was transforming my mind through persistent inner work. I never gave up on self-reflection or the commitment to grow into a more evolved version of myself. A major part of that work involved rewriting my inner narrative, which consisted of three interconnected practices: retelling, reframing, and releasing.

I had to retell the most painful story of my life, again and again, until I could see it clearly and compassionately. I told it until I knew in my bones that I was neither a victim nor a murderer, but an agent of change in my own life. I had to face the deep trauma of my brother's death and finally understand: it was not my fault.

As linguistic scholar Kathleen Ferrara noted in *Therapeutic Ways with Words*,[3] the stories we tell—and retell—within therapeutic settings don't just describe who we are; they help shape who we become. Rewriting my inner narrative wasn't just healing work, it was identity work.

Reframing followed naturally. I began to see that nothing is good or bad but thinking makes it so. Reframing didn't mean pretending it wasn't hard. It meant choosing to see my pain through a new lens—less as a punishment and more as a path. I shifted from asking "Why me?" to "What now?" From "What did I lose?" to "What have I gained?"

I stopped treating my past as a graveyard of failure and started treating it as fertile ground. In that shift, I began to rise—not in spite of my wounds, but through them.

And as I retold and reframed, I also had to release. I had to let go of the identity I had clung to, the one shaped by shame, survival, and silence, and also my academic identity, and I allowed something new to emerge in its place.

I had to loosen my grip on the academic persona I'd spent years building, the one that felt safe partly because it was praised and because I had pursued it for so many years. Letting go didn't happen all at once. But as I leaned more fully into writing and public speaking, I began to see that my true calling wasn't to lecture minds, but to tend souls—something I could never really do from behind the shield of academic distance.

5 Renewed My Mind by Training It to See the Positive

You have to train your mind to see the positive in everything—not in a fake, Pollyanna way, but in a determined, soul-saving way. I had to learn to turn over every scary-looking stone in my life to find the glints of beauty, meaning, or growth hiding underneath.

This wasn't a one-time shift; it was a moment-by-moment discipline, like weightlifting for the soul. I consciously converted grumbling into gratitude. I hunted joy. I interrogated every automatic negative thought. Over time, that repeated effort began to rewire my brain.

I was also fortunate to share space with my positive friend Lena. (It was, of course, a choice to welcome Lena and her optimism into my life—and to install her as a core member of my chosen family.) For the two years that I lived with her, we practiced the discipline of transforming every negative thought into something hopeful, humorous, or healing until it became natural.

Thus, changing every negative thought into something positive became my daily practice. Not in a way that denied pain, but in a way that refused to let it define me. Neuroplasticity is real. The more I chose hope, the easier it became to access.

I recently learned about Barbara Fredrickson's *Broaden-and-Build Theory*[4] of positive emotions, which perfectly explains how my intentional positivity grew into a sustained and flourishing happiness. According to her theory, positivity doesn't just feel good—it actually expands our awareness and builds long-term emotional resilience. Her theory suggests that positivity is cumulative and that it compounds over time.

That's exactly what happened in my life. The more I chose to see beauty, the more beautiful the world became. I didn't delete negative things from my life, I reinterpreted them. In this way, I feel that I redeemed them. I often withheld judgment like the Chinese farmer, musing "maybe so, maybe not." Thus, I not only reframed things, I also embraced impermanence and waited to see what positive things might rise in the wake of apparent loss. I watched my trauma torn brain slowly pivot toward peace, settle into presence, and begin to flirt with possibility.

6 Read Widely, Like My Soul Depended on It

Another major instrument of rewiring my brain (and reinforcing the positivity) was reading. I established the habit of reading over 100 books a year (about 85% of them now on audio). I read widely and deeply about healing, positivity, neuroplasticity, goal setting, spirituality and more. I also read uplifting fiction.

Reading has several wonderful effects. One, it significantly reduces stress. There's actually a study that shows that just reading for six minutes reduces stress by 68%, outperforming walking, music and tea![5]

Another study, commissioned by HarperCollins,[6] found something I've long suspected: people who identify as readers are more likely to describe themselves as "very happy." Among young adults, 40% of daily readers said they were very happy—compared to only 21% of non-readers. I believe that's because reading doesn't just entertain us—it shapes us. It gives us a language for longing, a mirror for our inner world, and sometimes, a ladder out of despair. Calling yourself a reader isn't just about how many books you finish—it's about how deeply you're letting stories help you live.

Whenever I got really upset and couldn't stop ruminating, I would read the *Outlander* series by Diana Gabaldon on audio. The series is full of love, spirituality, humor, and creativity. It helped me stop ruminating and rewire my brain to think positively when I was struggling. It's funny how we have the expression *garbage in, garbage out,* but we don't have its inverse, something like *gold in, gold out*. There it is, let's use it. Let's talk about it and let's do it.

When you fill your mind with goodness, knowledge, beauty, and truth, such will be the stuff that surges through your mind, such will be the fare that falls from your lips and flows from your life. Reading, especially deeply and reflectively, requires the brain to form and strengthen neural pathways. By reading deeply and widely, I am literally rewiring and transforming my mind.

7 Practiced Gratitude Continuously

I started a number of gratitude practices. I journaled about gratitude, I made long lists of things I was grateful for, I carried a stone around in my pocket, and every time I touched it, I expressed gratitude for something. I spent time meditating on what I am grateful for. I practiced being grateful not just for the obviously good things in my life but for the challenging things that had good outcomes hidden in their depths. I expressed gratitude for post-traumatic growth.

Psychologist Robert Emmons, one of the leading researchers on gratitude, has shown that consistent gratitude practice significantly boosts overall happiness, health, and life satisfaction[7]—and I found every bit of that to be true.

The habit I am most consistent with today is in my morning prayer and meditation time I spend a minimum of four minutes (but usually quite a bit more) expressing gratitude to God/the universe. However, it has become such a habit of thought that I am expressing gratitude in my mind and heart all day long. I continually stop and ask myself what beautiful things happened today, and I focus on and savor them.

It is my view that gratitude *is* happiness. Gratitude is literally just pausing to feel your happiness about elements of your life and expressing thankfulness about them.[8]

8 Set Goals

I also started setting goals like a crazy woman. Researcher Sonja Lyubomirsky has shown that setting and pursuing personally meaningful goals is one of the most effective strategies for increasing happiness—not because you always reach them, but because the pursuit itself fuels purpose, optimism, and well-being.[9] I often set 60 or 70 goals for a year. I'm not worried about not reaching all of them. If I reach 10 of them, I've won, but I usually reach far more than that. This has truly transformed my life.

There are two kinds of goals to set. One is a target of some kind (get a new job, participate in a speech contest). The other is establishing habits. Often, they go hand in hand. When I set a goal of reading 100 books in a year (a target goal), I set in motion a habit of reading constantly (a habit goal). Ultimately, it is our habits, more than our individual achievements, that transform us.

9 Served Others

Nine, I chose to serve others. For me, that meant joining the worship team at church as a lector, helping feed the unhoused, organizing a feeding program for Afghanistan, welcoming newly arrived immigrants, and mentoring others through Toastmasters. Whatever you can do to give to others will be a gamechanger. Just realizing you have something to give is a boon to your self-esteem.

There is substantial scientific research supporting the connection between altruism and happiness. There's actually something called the "helper's high,"[10] where your brain releases feel-good chemicals like dopamine, oxytocin and endorphins when you engage in prosocial activity. Multiple studies show that people who regularly volunteer or help others report greater overall life satisfaction and lower rates of depression. This was very much my experience.

10 Reveled in Creativity

Finally, the tenth ingredient for me was creativity. I reminded myself of my strengths in writing and speaking, and I started setting goals related to those strengths. For me, that meant writing a lot. First, I wrote a children's chapter book about positivity and inclusion called *This Little Pig is Family*. Then I wrote 100 poems in one year, developed several blogs, and presented a lot of speeches (which I first had to write). Even praying for people after the service at church was an act of creativity.

Psychologist Mihaly Csikszentmihalyi describes creativity as one of the most direct paths to joy, because it brings us into a state of flow—a kind of joyful absorption where time disappears and meaning expands.[11] All this creativity was enjoyable in its own right, but it also gave joy to others, and giving joy to others gave even more joy to me.

Choose Your Tools and Rebuild

Everything I've shared here is a window into what worked for me—not a prescription, but a witness. Just to recap, here is the shortlist:

1. Obtained psychiatric care, trauma informed therapist

2. Established community

3. Developed a spiritual practice

4. Rewrote my inner narrative

5. Transformed my mind re: positivity

6. Read like my soul depended on it

7. Practiced gratitude continuously

8. Set lots of goals

9. Served others

10. Reveled in creativity

These weren't magic steps. In the beginning they were daily, clumsy, hopeful choices I kept making until my life began to take shape again. As I read more, they became more strategic. Your resurrection will not look like mine. But I believe that whatever ashes you're rising from, you too have access to tools—maybe even these same ones. You are not powerless. You are not done. The road is long, but transformation is real. Choose your tools. Begin again. You get to build the life you want to live inside.

---

1. Waldinger, Robert, and Marc Schulz. *The Good Life: Lessons from the World's Longest Scientific Study of Happiness*. Simon & Schuster, 2023.

2. Lyubomirsky, Sonja. *The How of Happiness: A New Approach to Getting the Life You Want*. Penguin, 2007.

3. Ferrara, Kathleen. *Therapeutic Ways with Words*. Oxford University Press, 1994.

4. Fredrickson, Barbara. *Positivity: Groundbreaking Research Reveals How to Embrace the Hidden Strength of Positive Emotions, Overcome Negativity, and Thrive.* Crown Publishers, 2009.

5. Lewis, David. "Galaxy Stress Research." *Mindlab International, University of Sussex,* 2009, as cited in "Reading Reduces Stress. Fact.," *Medicine in Literature,* 19 Jan. 2023

6. HarperCollins UK. "New research reveals that 29% of 14–25 year olds strongly think of themselves as a reader, with significant benefits to their mental health." *HarperCollins UK,* 2024.

7. Emmons, Robert A. *Thanks!: How the New Science of Gratitude Can Make You Happier.* Houghton Mifflin, 2007.

8. I am aware that gratitude scientists will parse these into separate experiences and I'm ok with that.

9. Lyubomirsky, Sonja. *The How of Happiness: A New Approach to Getting the Life You Want.* Penguin Press, 2007.

10. Post, Stephen G. "It's Good to Be Good: 2011 Fifth Annual Scientific Report on Health, Happiness and Helping Others." *International Journal of Person Centered Medicine,* vol. 1, no. 4, 2011, pp. 814–829.

11. Csikszentmihalyi, Mihaly. *Creativity: Flow and the Psychology of Discovery and Invention.* Harper Perennial, 1997.

20

— • —

TAKING CANCER'S KEYS

Just when I had begun to live my life out loud, radiant and reveling in joy, the unimaginable happened. After nearly a decade of clawing my way out of my own spiritual grave, standing triumphantly on the mountain I made out of a hole (instead of a mole hill), I found myself standing face to face with that raggedy assed rat bastard, The Grim Reaper, in the form of Stage IV Pancreatic Cancer. Talk about a plot twist.

What Grim didn't know, bless his little black shriveled up heart, was that I was so full of life that even death could not destroy me. I was prepared to die if I must, and to do so with strength and beauty. I was not afraid.

(Quick note to readers who might be in the thick of it now, this might be one to come back to in pieces. Read what you can. Skip what you don't need now. I trust you. And remember I am just reporting from the trenches—my trenches. I'm not trying to challenge anyone else's experience. I can imagine situations where my response is not possible or not desirable.)

Once I learned how to take control of my own narrative, I was prepared to take away cancer's keys. When cancer came into your life, either to you or to a loved one, especially if it was your first confrontation with cancer, you may have felt like you completely lost control of the wheel. I'm not sure you would be human if you felt otherwise. The question is, does losing some control mean you have lost all control? Can you take the wheel back? And if so, how?

How Diane's Cancer Journey and My Resurrection Prepared Me for My Own Cancer

When Diane died, cancer absolutely hijacked my life and wrecked it thoroughly, and I let myself get dragged along for the ride. But the process was highly educational. Fool me once, shame on you... well, there the shame will stay because it won't be happening a second time (let's not count that early childhood mess).

This time cancer probably thought that she would be driving again, bully that she is, but I decided I own this life, and I am taking back the keys. I'm driving! You can get in the back seat. Cancer happened to me, and I can't wave my magic wand and drive it away, but it's not completely hijacking my story.

I decided that even if cancer forced me to a premature end, it was not taking over my story. It doesn't have to be a unilateral affair. Cancer may happen to me, but I can also happen to cancer! Watch me. I hear my mother's voice in my head, "Hide and watch," (finally that energy was back!)

I decided this story wasn't going to descend on me and confine and define me. I decided to take charge of it. I couldn't choose all the events, but I could choose my response to those events and my interpretation of the significance of those events. And there were many events I *could* choose, while there were others I could shape and direct.

If I had not journeyed through the shadow of death with Diane, I don't know how I would have told my cancer story to myself. But because I had achieved my healing and because this was not my first rodeo, I was ready. If cancer catches you totally unaware, it will suck a lot of soul energy away, forcing you to sort out all your existential stuff, figure out your preferences for managing the disease, make decisions about end-of-life actions in case they are necessary, and all of that on top of fighting for your life every day. Unless, perhaps, you can borrow preparation from someone else's story.

Fortuitously, I had worked out ninety percent of that stuff through my experience with Diane. I didn't have to waste any time sorting through the philosophical and spiritual questions a death sentence usually evokes (I have included my personal answers to these questions in the chapters ahead, so that you might benefit from my experience if you like). I knew exactly how I would manage my cancer journey. I knew what I wanted from my loved ones. I knew what I wanted from myself.

Diane's cancer journey was a hell of a ride, as was my long inner healing journey in its aftermath, but at the end of that time, I emerged a person full of joy and love and positivity. And being that healthy, whole person prepared me to weather the storm of my life.

I still had to deal with a few relationships that needed ironing out, and I still had to make end-of-life decisions about burial, funeral, property, and what would happen to my writing. But for the most part, I had the hard stuff all squared away. And that freed me to be very positive and proactive about my own cancer experience.

Seven Keys I Specifically Took Back

I didn't write them down at the time, but looking back, I can see that I made seven resolutions about my cancer journey that made all the difference.

First of all, there is more light in me than there is darkness in cancer. I decided to radiate light and blast the gloom. I decided I'm going to shine on my story, I'm going to shine on my body, I'm going to shine on my loved ones, I'm going to shine on everyone I come in contact with. I am full of light and I defy the darkness! You can. not. extinguish. me. I defy you!

Second, I was born to love. I am going to pour out as much love on others as I can possibly squeeze out of my soul in whatever time I have left. My last chapter will be my last act of love. Cancer will not deter me from my purpose.

Third, I am going to take advantage of my ultimate teachable moments. I am a teacher to the bone, and I always wanted to write about grief and help people process better than I had because nobody should have their life wrecked for twenty years or fifty years by grief (and yet it happens all the time). I wanted to help other people manage grief better.

Grief wrecks us. The more someone has grown into our souls, the harder it is to lose them—it's like they are being ripped out, and part of our soul comes out with them. It feels like an amputation of some part of our core that can never be replaced and feels like it will never heal. What I want to shout to the world is that healing happens! My life is proof. You have to fight for it. It doesn't come easily. Its pursuit is not for the faint of heart. But I believe healing does happen. It is attainable.

I found myself facing my own imminent demise and thinking that I had lost my opportunity. But then I realized this could *be* my opportunity. One of the things I could do with my last chapter is help my loved ones grieve. I'm good at grieving. Maybe I can show you how to do it more efficiently than I did before. I love the idea that I might teach right up to my dying breath.

Fourth, I am going to spend more time feeling grateful for each joy in my life than I am going to spend moaning about what hurts. Joy and grief grow up together. They are not mutually exclusive. I am the one who determines my focus.

Other people can manage their cancer as it seems best to them. I am not prescribing gratitude, but as for me and myself, I choose to elevate joy and love and beauty to the best of my ability. I will let myself feel the pain. I will let myself grieve. But I am not going to let grief drown out the beauty in my life.

Fifth, cancer may make me cry, but she can't stop me from laughing. Humor lifts your own attitude; it's powerful. It gives you control over your feelings and also some interactional power. It also builds solidarity and relationship. You need community. Part of your community will be the healthcare professionals you spend so much time with. Brighten their lives and you will brighten your own. A little strategically inserted humor here and there will help.

Is humor the ultimate reframing tool? If not the opposite of fear, it is certainly a fierce opponent of fear. Humor is a way of savoring the moment. It is a way of focusing on NOW. It's about joy eclipsing sorrow. As I noted in the beginning of this book, when you see humor in the situation, you take the power away from circumstances and show life who's boss. Laughter really is good for the soul. And what's good for the soul is usually good for the body as well. Anything you view with humor can spice up your life. Humor is driven by hope and defiance. I shall embrace it at every opportunity.

Sixth, I want to be intentional about the close of each relationship. A very important part of me lives on in the hearts and memories of those who knew and loved me. Closing that relationship lovingly is my last gift to them. It merits my full attention.

I shall be intentional. I will ask for forgiveness. I will offer forgiveness. I will acknowledge the good I see—I will not die with undisclosed praise or affection in me. I will offer whatever wisdom I may have acquired and give my best advice. I will endeavor not to manipulate or ask for anything impossible.

I want to help my loved ones grieve by not leaving open wounds in them. I think I can be a healer even as I die. I will plan my face-to-face but also leave them something in writing that they can return to again and again, something a little more permanent than that last ephemeral conversation. Poems, letters, journals, songs, scrapbook pages. Photos. Sacred objects, videos. I want to leave them something tangible.

Finally, seventh, reframing. Cancer is not running the show. I'm in charge and I will define my health, myself and my situation as I see fit. I will reframe everything about these circumstances according to my own preferences.

Those are seven keys I took back from cancer, and I think I can recommend them.

Real Time Dispatches from the Frontline

The last section of this book is made up mostly of real time blog posts I made while standing in the whirlwind of the stage IV diagnosis. They are messier, more immediate, raw. Sometimes repetitive. Sometimes perhaps too sharp or too soft. But they are real. They are true. And truth, whether messy or not, is holy ground.

I wanted you to see the dates and understand my process in responding to my diagnosis on May 22, 2020. I had to review some of the existential riddles that had first come up when Diane died and decide whether they still fit or not. Most of them did. Some coalesced in the presence of this diagnosis in a way they had not during Diane's passing. Perhaps some of my conclusions will be helpful to you.

21

—·—

HAVING A LITTLE CHAT WITH "BOB" (AND THEN MY PEEPS)

It was a gorgeous day in May when they told me I had, perhaps, a year to live. The world did not shatter. The birds continued to sing. The sun, oblivious, poured out light on the evil and the good. I still had terrible stomach pain, and they told me not to eat anything for x number of hours, but I felt I owed myself a strawberry shake for dragging myself to ER, so I stopped for one.

I then proceeded to get lost driving home on a well-known route. My head was full of psycho-static and I was talking to my pastor on the phone and just couldn't manage the multitask. Oh, and it was during the covid lockdown, so I couldn't just go see anyone I wanted and get a hug. There was a lot going on.

I did not rage or plead or collapse in a heap. Instead, I had a little talk with the cosmos— with "Bob," the universe, God, or whatever cosmic committee was running the show—and asked what the hell kind of plot twist this was. I was just getting good at being alive. This made no sense (a concept you'd think I would have gotten used to by now).

This chapter is not a textbook case. It's a dispatch from the deep interior, a field note scribbled in the margins of a diagnosis, where grief and wonder, absurdity and grace, held hands and waited to see what I'd do next.

Everybody Thinks They Know the Stages of Grief

It seems that almost everyone "knows" about the five stages of grief popularized by Elisabeth Kübler-Ross[1] in the 1960s (Denial, Anger, Bargaining, Depression, and Acceptance).

There has been so much progress in the area of Thanatology (that's the study of death, dying, and bereavement) beyond the idea of stages in the fifty years since she essentially founded the field, but ironically, the idea of five immutable stages will not die.

This idea has made it so far into our cultural consciousness that it shows up in memes about silly things like spilled coffee and failed Zoom calls. However, most people have not actually read about her work and don't really understand what Kübler-Ross intended and the ways her stages have been misapplied.

The first common misunderstanding is the belief that she was writing about the grief that the living experience when they lose a loved one. In fact, she was originally writing about the experience of the person who was dying and coming to terms with their own death. Her book was based on interviews with 200 dying people and identified the patterns that she saw in those interviews (a relatively small number to generalize to seven or eight billion people).

The second misunderstanding is the belief that everyone experiences all five stages. Actually, you might never experience some of the stages.

The third misunderstanding is that there is a predetermined sequence of these states of mind and you channel through them sequentially, one after another—and just once. In fact, you may not experience all five stages, you may experience stages over and over, and they can happen in any order and even simultaneously. Grief is just not all modular and linear like that.

It's my guess that the people most committed to this model are people who haven't had to struggle with grief on a large scale yet. And the big problem with these misunderstandings is that they give people on the outside the false confidence that they know what you're going through and how fast and in what order you should be going through it.

They may step in to give you unsolicited and unearned advice. They may put your grief on a timetable. They may criticize you for not evidencing all of the stages (like anger, for instance). It's OK for you to politely tell them to go fly a kite.

Mild Outrage at "Bob"

It is true that a very common response to having your life or that of someone you love threatened is that of rage. That's why Kübler-Ross included it in her model—because it was a common response. It is not, however, a mandatory stage. Not everyone experiences it every time they face a loss.

In fact, looking back, I don't think I have ever experienced anger as a stage of grief. I imagine this is because I first encountered death when I was four. My mother also reports that she did not experience anger as a part of her early agony. When the doctor told me I had a year to live, I was not angry either. I think my prior experience with grief caused me to go straight to acceptance and the deep grief of knowing I was losing every single person I loved by losing myself.

Have you ever heard that delightful Southern gospel song, *Have a Little Talk with Jesus?* It's worth YouTubing (Dolly Parton has a lovely version).[2] I have heard plenty of atheists mention having little conversations with the universe or whatever externalized mysterious force might be out there after all—pulling unseen strings and manipulating terrestrial outcomes in times of duress, so I don't think the experience is peculiar to a variety of evangelical (and again, I do not currently identify as one, but I was whelped by them).

On my way home from the ER, I had a little chat with "Bob." My first response to this grim diagnosis was, *WTF? I had the next sixty years planned out! I was going to be a star! I was going to redeem the lameness of the last fifty years with the next! I was going to be rich and famous!* Well, mostly I was going to spread healing to the world, but if a modicum of success came to me along the way that would have been swell.

And I just lost fifty pounds! For what? So I can look skinny in my casket? That was not even on my bucket list! I haven't been this hot in years, and for what?? Anyway, I'm going to be cremated—nobody will even notice my tiny waist! I am never going to find the love of my life now. Doesn't matter. Might as well be ugly and fat.

I got a PhD that took me a hundred years to finalize! I got almost all my wounds healed! Who does that? I did! And why? So I could go and effin' die? Might as well be dysfunctional and wounded beyond belief, drinking myself into oblivion in Margaritaville! What was the point of all this painstaking, heartbreaking, grueling work on myself??

I have finally become happy. I have finally come to love my life and myself in just the last year. What? I get one year of happiness? (Well sure, I maybe had ten if I pieced them all together, but that was the first really happy year in twenty). If the universe does have a plan, it's a stupid one. This doesn't make any sense.

It would be fair to characterize my feelings as severe shock accompanied by mild-to-moderate outrage. It didn't feel like anger, just hard-core indignation.

Oh, That Damned River in Egypt, De-nial

But I was not in denial. I don't remember ever having that experience with death or grief, either, even when I was younger. I historically do not do denial (except maybe for that one little detail of Brian).

I have been a straight shooter from the get-go. If you want the unvarnished truth, I'm your girl. Ok, I've gotten slightly better with varnish over time, but I don't pretend. Authenticity is my brand. As my friend Abe graciously said, I have a way of getting straight to the heart of the matter. Born that way. Then forged in the fire of life events that would rip any lingering naïveté away for good. I tell it like it is, keep it real, make no bones about it, mince no words and religiously avoid sugar coating. I have learned to be gentle about it, but clear.

First of all, I just know from hanging around that there are some cancers where people simply die swiftly. When Diane was diagnosed with stomach cancer in 1999, everyone I had ever known who had stomach cancer died in three to six months.

And second, I didn't go into denial about people dying after I had that firsthand experience of watching someone I loved more than life die a hellish death. God—it didn't have to be as hellish as it was. All the chemo and cutting just made the last chapter of her life grim and gruesome.

Sinister state governments do not devise "enhanced interrogation" methods as horrific as the things we sometimes do trying to save some scrap of quantity of the life of a cancer patient that will have no quality. I don't think she would have agreed to all those hellish treatments if she had not been in denial about how advanced her cancer was.

I, on the other hand, when I was diagnosed with late-stage pancreatic cancer, had no delusions about what was ahead of me. I could not know the particularities, but I knew the basic terrain. I had had two decades to contemplate the meaning of my life and work out all those existential riddles ahead of time that most people don't really face until their own number is up. I congratulated myself on CLEPing out of Death and Dying 101, 111, and 112. I had had the benefit of Advanced Placement Death Education. More time for electives, you know.

Getting This Show on the Road

So, I hit the ground running. I assembled my amazing care team (to be fair I commissioned them and then they assembled themselves like a well-oiled machine) and I got busy immediately plotting out the course, with their assistance.

Planning for the completion of your life is like planning a wedding, so many moving parts, so many things that have to be done in a certain order. Many people die unnecessarily untidy deaths and leave so many strings untied. This is no gift to the loved ones who remain to do the tying, or to live the rest of their lives without closure.

When I got home, I started packing my stuff away to make my room invalid-friendly. As I reorganized my space, I tried to organize my thoughts. I was trying to determine how close I could get my bed to the bathroom. How could I make more space for chairs around my bed so my friends could hang out?

I packed away almost all of my books. *What's the point of reading? It's not like I'm ever going to use this brain for anything else again. What is the point of the treadmill? It's not like I'm going to have this heart much longer.* For a day or two, I felt the utter futility of daily activities.

Happy Birthday, Mom

The day I was diagnosed was actually my mother's birthday. My brother, Eric, had died just two and a half years prior, suddenly at age forty-seven. My other brother had died in childhood. My mother had had four children and by the time of my diagnosis, two had already died. I hurt for her almost more than myself. I wanted to wait a few days to tell her.

One of my dearest friends is a psychotherapist. When I suggested that I should wait a few days to tell my mother the news, she was adamant, "You do not have the right to decide how much someone else can handle. Furthermore, you are probably more worried about what *you* can handle." She is a very wise woman, and I saw that she was right.

Resigning myself, I sucked it up and called my mom on her birthday to tell her that I was going to die soon. And I'm glad I did. My mom was heartbroken, but she is a tough old bird. She has known far more suffering than I have, and that's saying something. That was such an important lesson for me to learn, and I am so grateful to my friend for teaching it to me. It is patronizing and paternalistic to decide what someone else can handle. I couldn't be that person.

My closest friends came over that night to hang out on the deck. We were already gathering to celebrate my birthday late. I didn't want to do it back in April because I wanted to be able to help my friend who was having surgery, so I was super self-isolating from Covid. It was a glorious spring day. Just beautiful. So, we ended up celebrating my birthday on the day I found out my death day was imminent.

I checked with my friend, Maranda, who owns the house my apartment was in, to make sure she didn't mind me dying under her roof. She graciously agreed. Everything was coming together smoothly.

Surprise Discovery About Myself (I Am Not Afraid)

I was extremely surprised to find that I did not feel afraid of dying or even of suffering. I felt afraid of not having enough time to do this well. To tie up every relationship I had as beautifully as I could. I was afraid I wouldn't have time to impress upon each beloved just how much I loved them. Ideally, I would like to write each one of them an epic poem, among other things. My Muse is slow as molasses, however, and I knew I didn't have time for that.

Now the question is, even if you begin with acceptance and you dive right into the hard work of getting stuff done to plan for the eventual probable outcome, if you are not crushed and in utter despair, does that mean you're still in some level of denial? I have had way more crushing in my life than any one person should... I feel like I've been run over by a steamroller repeatedly. Isn't it possible that I just knew that I would survive this?

I know how ridiculous it sounds to speak of surviving death even though you fully anticipate experiencing it (and I'm pretty amused by the image). I mean, this is not unthinkable. It is totally thinkable. Look! I am thinking it now! Your head will not explode by contemplating and accepting this generally undesired outcome. But as I said, I have known since early childhood that one's number can be up at any single point on the continuum of your potential life. And I feel so blessed that my number was this high. I have lived a lot!

I cried periodically throughout the day. But it was not my default state. My default state was joy. I wondered if this joy-laced grief was some special subspecies of denial I had not read about. Was my positive attitude a kind of denial even though I was furiously making plans to die?

We would only know, I decided, as we watched this journey unfold. I promised to try not to be devastated if I found out that there is some predictable human pattern of behavior that I was experiencing and later found myself in despair at some point along the way.

Getting Overwhelmed by Other People's Grief

If you had (or have) cancer, who would end up with the job of telling everyone else? Do you want to do that yourself or are you ok outsourcing the task to others so you can focus on the work at hand? No judgment one way or the other. I found out I was very hands-on in that regard.

If you do decide to do it yourself, I think you will find that coming out to people about your cancer is, for a few weeks, a full-time job. I feel the need to take care of all of them. That first week, I wasn't able to even think about my classes or my grades. I needed to be able to compartmentalize, to carve out cancer-free blocks in my schedule to get stuff done.

As an empath, I can get so overwhelmed by other people's emotions. I remember when I was younger, I would feel totally crushed under the weight of everyone else's suffering. Someone (usually some man) would ask me what was wrong, and when I listed everything that was weighing on me, he would look at me quizzically and say, "But none of that is happening to you. Those are other people's problems." I was as mystified by his perspective as he was by mine. Although I had plenty of trauma and suffering of my own, I felt I also managed to carry the pain of just about everyone I loved inside, too...

So, when it came time to tell everyone about my death sentence, I had to do it little by little because I could only absorb so much pain at a time. And once I had told my mother, I could start telling everyone else. I wanted to tell them myself. I didn't want the most important news of my life to just fly out on the grapevine like cheap gossip. I wanted to tell my dearest ones one-on-one. I asked all of them to keep it to themselves until I was ready for it to be made public. And they honored that.

I felt the emotional weight of loving so many people so deeply and had these wonderful intimate deep conversations with dear ones all over the world—in Japan, Korea, Germany, Belgium, Spain. Thank God for the miracle of the internet! (Note to self: telling someone on Zoom that you're going to die is exponentially harder than doing so on the phone).

I know it was my grief over losing them as much as feeling their grief. It was overwhelming. My brain darted around in a thousand directions, and it was super hard to focus on next steps. I was trying to think who I had to tell next, before telling whom. I felt the order was critical. I wanted some control over the unfolding narrative that was going out.

And for the most part, all those conversations were beautiful. Grief only exists because of love. It is often said that grief is the price of love and that's true. If you don't want the pain of grief, you can choose not to love anyone. And some people, tragically, do make that choice. They don't get attached because they don't want to experience loss. Thus, they experience the greater loss of never having the richness of intimacy and deep love in their lives.

For me, the beautiful part of this experience of breaking the news to my dear ones was all the love that was expressed between us in those interactions. Love flowed as profusely as our tears.

My niece, Teresa, had fainted when she learned that her dad (my brother, Eric) had died, so when I called her with my news, I made her go into a quiet room and sit down before I told her. I asked one of my favorite cousins if she would please tell my dear Uncle Jim (I could not bear to tell him), who lost his wife twenty-five years ago, has no children, and considers me his kid. He has been like a doting father to me. This is what he texted me: "ALL MY LOVE, TO ELISA!!!! I love your guts!!!![3] Starting on my tomato cages, now." My friend Dee chuckled when I read the text to her. "Whatever helps you grieve, Uncle Jim. Tomatoes it is."

My friend Ashley said, "I don't know what to say. You taught me love." She could not have said anything more soothing to my heart. My friend Anna said, "You taught us love and beauty and how to live." Well, that was an unexpected gift rising out of our grief.

Getting By with a Little Help from My Friends

So many friends threatened to hop on a plane and come see me. To which I replied, "Stay the %$## away! If I get covid with cancer, I will die a swift and horrible death and that is not how I want to go out." I asked them to send me stuffed animals as stand ins for hugs and write me love letters instead. I got several love letters from family that mean the world to me.

Brendon Burchard asks himself at the end of every day, "Did I live, did I love, did I matter?"[4] What I wanted most to hear from my loved ones was that I had made their lives better in some way, had loved them, had brought some modicum of healing or helped them think about how they could love each other better. I found so much peace from the flood of responses like these that came in. It was tremendously gratifying.

My mom called the next morning to remind me to play the guitar (don't get excited, I am a terrible guitar player) because it always comforts me. Of course, she did not use the word *comfort*. That would be way too touchy-feely. But it was so kind and uncharacteristic. She prefers to avoid negative emotions. But she let me know that she sees me (blindness notwithstanding) and she does know how sensitive I am, and she does know what helps me. I don't know how to say what a gift that was to me.

My sister kindly contacted the cemetery where my father and my two brothers are buried to see if there was a plot available. They said there was a spot open there, and they don't keep records past twenty-three years, so they didn't know if it had been paid for, but it was only twenty dollars! (It's in a very small town in Kansas). Then they called my sister back and decided it had already been paid for.

I think they probably thought, "Geez, these people are dying off like flies. Maybe we should give them a buy three-get-one-free friends and family discount." I felt really good about being able to be buried with my family. Besides, that section of the graveyard needed some female representation.

Yes, I Want to Live

By the morning of Day Four, I had already broken the hearts of most of my loved ones by breaking the news. I was already divvying up my belongings among my loved ones in my head, making lists of things I needed to do to wind up financial obligations.

I was also congratulating myself on all the sucky things I would miss out on by not growing old (you know, student loans, watching your face shrivel up like a prune, facing that painful day when someone takes your driver's license and keys away, and that other painful day when the doctor tells you to stop climbing trees, as happened to my Aunt Alice merely because she fell out of one when she was seventy).

I began to realize that a lot of people were dismayed that I assumed I would be coming to completion very soon with advanced metastatic pancreatic cancer. I mean, seriously, every time they looked inside me, they found new "masses," which is of course code for *tumor*, thus proving them to be liberally distributed throughout my body (at one point I had over 18 tumors and disease sites including bone marrow involvement and they had stopped counting. They just said, "You have a LOT of disease.")

A few people asked me, "Do you even want to live?" Oh my God, I want to live! But I am a realist. Some cancers are swift at stage four. I understand this to be one of them.[5] My sweet friend was in denial until the final weeks of her life and, as a consequence, her death was messy and kind of disastrous. I didn't want my final chapter to be like that. I wanted it to be well-written. I wanted to tidy all of my affairs and leave all of my loved ones with closure in our relationships. I wanted to help them grieve, if I could.

I realized a few days in, however, when talking to my friend Stacy (who was an oncology nurse for many years), that my view of cancer treatment was really stuck in 2001 when I watched Diane die. I realized there might be treatments that would not destroy the quality of my life, and I am totally open to that kind of treatment.

Yes, I would still prefer to live to 120, so if there are treatments that could make that happen, I would obviously be ecstatic. I just never want my life extended where I'm stuck in a hospital bed looking like a corpse already with a tube down my nose and wounds that won't heal, vomiting all over my tubes every few minutes. I have already done that vicariously. It was almost worse than the "saved life" of Khal Drogo in *Game of Thrones*. That kind of extension of life is not welcome. There are fates worse than death. Life is so much more than not being dead.

I want to be loving people up to the last minute of my life. I find that harder to do when in agony. And it's also harder for those who have to see me suffer to receive love in those circumstances. I didn't want that.

So, I told them, "Let's just see what's available and play it by ear. I choose life, but that means actual life. Not artificial, barely alive "life.""

Y'all choose what's best for you. As for me and myself, we ain't doing that.

---

1. Kübler-Ross, Elisabeth. *On Death and Dying*. Macmillan, 1969.

2. *"Dolly Parton Performs 'Just a Little Talk with Jesus' with Natalie Grant." YouTube*, uploaded by *Dollymania* (or the original uploader, if known), 11 Mar. 2023, http://www.youtube.com/watch?v=T%E2%80%91sLN22F6gY .

3. When I was a teenager, I used to tell everyone I loved their guts—you know, it's basic synecdoche, referring to a part to indicate the whole.

4. Burchard, Brendon. *The Charge: Activating the 10 Human Drives That Make You Feel Alive*. Free Press, 2012.

5. I guess a year is not that swift as cancers go, but it felt swift to me.

The Joy of Loving Me

Enveloped by My Chosen Bonus Family

As I (perhaps nauseatingly) noted before, by the time of my diagnosis, my life was overflowing with love. I had so many loving communities, and I especially had a little knot of chosen bonus family who are truly the siblings of my soul.

So even though I was physically alone on the day I received my diagnosis in the ER, my friends were all texting me throughout and Dee, perhaps the bravest among us, called me immediately when I reported my diagnosis. I felt surrounded by love. I truly felt that they were right there with me.

Of my closest friends, Tina, Dayna, and Andre all lost their mothers when they themselves were in their twenties. Mike lost his father to cancer later, and Maranda's sister is a lymphoma survivor. Tina and Vickie are survivors, and Dee was believed to have ovarian cancer in her twenties until surgery revealed otherwise. Only one of my closest friends, Lena, has not had such an experience with cancer, and I think that might be why she took my diagnosis the hardest. She couldn't even talk to me about it for quite some time. Moreover, all of my friends are nurturing, giving people with lots of caregiving experience. It was like I had won the friend lottery. I was lavished upon.

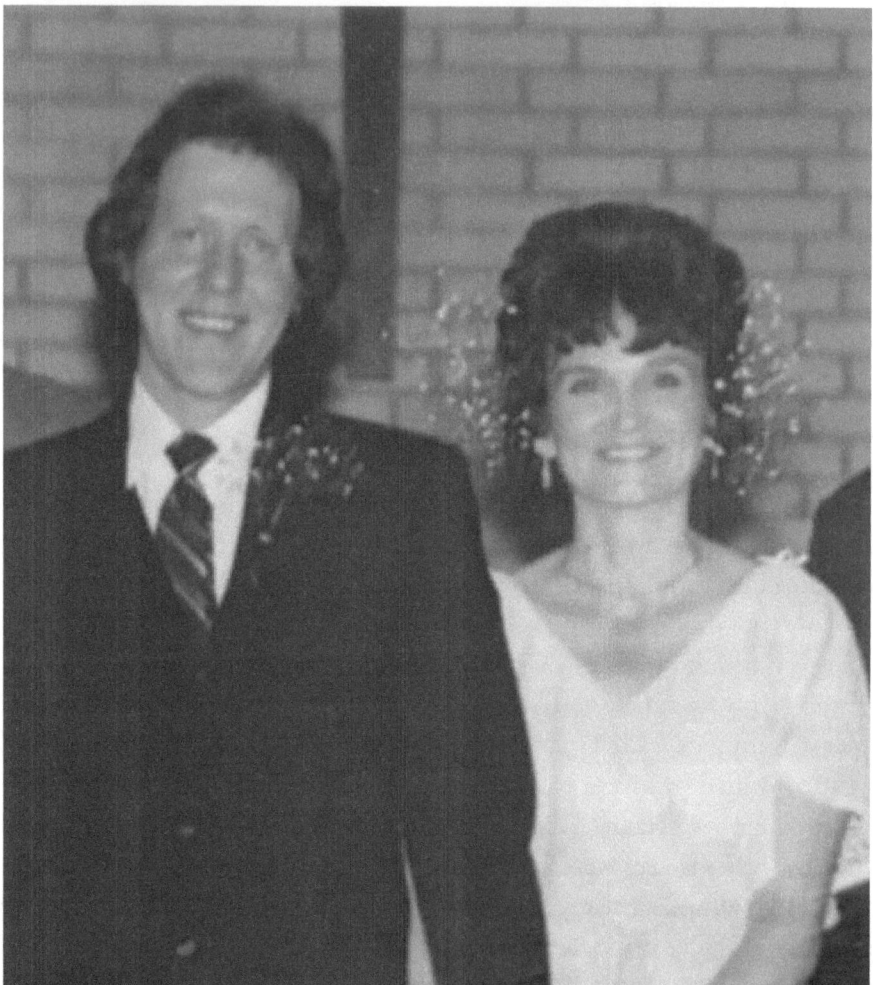

Gail and Mom on their wedding day 1981

Having the Grace to Let You Be My Servant, Too

If you have never had any experience with caregiving (from either side), you may not have developed any preferences or thought about how you'd like to be treated in a situation where you needed to be on the receiving end.

Being the oldest child of a blind woman is not *exactly* a caregiving position, but it is one where you must be very attuned to assisting someone else. My mother is a fiercely independent woman, one you do not want to make the mistake of patronizing. I grew up very sensitive to and very aware of the delicate affair of trying to help people without making them feel that they are being helped, without compromising their own independent identities.

Of course, Americans are almost pathologically addicted to their independence and a lot more likely to get their nose out of joint over an offer of help than people from many other cultures.

I became even more sensitive to this when I studied my mother's interactions with her sighted companions for my dissertation. Honestly, it used to really irritate me how my mother would slowly make her way through the house to bring my stepfather his tea, seemingly forty times a day. I always thought, *Why can't you go get your own damned tea? It will take you a quarter of the time.* She even ironed his shirts (my mom and I would go round and round about whether blind people should iron. I think you can guess who won those rounds).

But when I finally let myself take off all my psychological insulation and think about her situation, I realized that, of the two of us, it was I who was the blinder.

Not My Cup of Tea

One thing my mother loved was riding the Honda Goldwing she and my stepfather owned, and he drove her all over the Midwest on that thing on their vacations. (If you imagine that I objected even more to the motorcycle than the iron, you imagine right).

When I was studying blind/sighted interaction for my research, it occurred to me that I didn't know how she manages public bathrooms now that neither I nor my sister are constantly by her side to help her. How does she know the stall is empty, that there's nobody scary in there, that every surface she is about to come in contact with is clean, how does she get oriented to each new bathroom and so on?

When I asked her, it turns out that Gail (my stepfather) would go into a McDonald's, for example, and explain, "My wife is blind and needs me to assist her in the bathroom; can you go in and make sure it's clear for me to do so?" This is only one of the many extraordinary ways he helped her every single day, always without making her feel that she was being helped.

And I finally understood the tea. And the ironing and the cooking and every other thing she did for him. It's all about balance and making sure this was a symmetrical relationship where each gave to the other equally. In a loving relationship, you serve each other.

And just because I think it's too much to ask a blind person to do something a sighted person can do with a fraction of the effort does not mean I get to decide what she thinks is too much trouble to do for someone else. How could I be so patronizing?

And how could I fail to see what an extraordinary soul he was for being able to mediate the visual world for her without ever making her feel beholden to him? Gail had this uncanny ability to master the ecology of interability discourse. You need empathy, but you must have equal parts respect. Without respect, empathy deteriorates into sympathy, and nobody with a disability of any kind wants that.

There is a beautiful hymn written by a New Zealander named Richard Gillard that asks, "Will you let me be your servant, let me be as Christ to you? Pray that I might have the grace to let you be my servant, too." For over forty years, my stepfather quietly served her and had the grace to let her be his servant, too.

PSA: What I Need Emotionally and Psychologically

As for me and my own caregiving community, I immediately started a Google Drive Document to communicate with my care team of closest friends. Having witnessed more than enough of what I did not want, I felt it was necessary to lay out my ground rules and philosophy of this caregiving relationship from the get-go. I realize not everyone has a philosophy of caregiving because not everyone has had the experience and the opportunity to ruminate about it, but over the course of five decades, I had.

I learned that people are not mind-readers, and you cannot blame them for that. You have to educate them about your needs and wishes. Community and relationship are collaborative dances. You have to do your part. And if you have more experience with this situation, even if you are in the hot seat and are the one needing care, you have more responsibility for educating your loved ones.

This is what I sent them the day after my diagnosis:

How I Feel about All of You

May 23, 2020

The most important thing you need to know is how deeply loved I feel by all of you and how comforted I am to know that I do not walk this path alone. I feel enveloped by your love. I cannot imagine anyone having a more loving family of friends surrounding and supporting them than I have in you. Also, I have arrived at a state of sufficient self-love and self-compassion and multilateral grace that I can acknowledge that loving me is as much a joy to you as loving you is to me.

What I Ask from You

Obviously, one of the most awful things about being seriously ill (or having a disability) is the deep sense of powerlessness that overtakes you. First, you are powerless because you can't change your situation, and you can't predict what's going to happen when. So, there is a loss of control inherent in the physical, existential condition.

But there is another kind of powerlessness that can be avoided. Well-meaning loved ones may feel that it is their place to give and the other person's place to receive, unilaterally. I need you to let me continue giving to you as long as I can. I need for you to let me feel that there is still some interdependence among us. That I am not merely the helpless recipient of your loving care. I will *be* the gracious recipient of your loving care, but I need to have the agency to also give to you in whatever ways I am able.

Also, I know that I am not responsible for your emotions, but do not begrudge me the desire to protect you or comfort you. I have learned (through certain people's insistence, ahem) that I don't get to decide how much you can handle (and sometimes that's more about how much I can handle), so I won't hide anything from you. But I also get to be compassionate.

Furthermore, my body may be broken, but I am NOT AN EMOTIONAL INVALID. I do have a psychological and emotional mountain to scale. But I'm kind of an emotional triathlete. Please do not break my heart by suddenly becoming unable to receive my love or letting me love you in whatever way I can. Loving you is an anchor in this ever-looming cloud formation that threatens to unleash a torrent of apparent futility on me. (I know this metaphor is imperfect! I plead cognitive psychostatic).

I need your compassion, but I also need your continued admiration. I need the satisfaction of knowing that I have something beautiful to offer you. Is that selfish enough for you? I need you to resist the temptation to view me as moving into a state of being an emotional invalid. I really need you to see me as an emotional triathlete who has been training for this contest all my life. I will practice self-compassion, I promise. And I know you will help me stay on track with that.

My Philosophy of My Pain vs. My Independence

These are my decisions for now. I am not an invalid yet. And I am definitely not feeble minded. I have an excellent brain, an excellent decision-making ability, and I am extremely responsible. I know when I am in my right mind.

I will continue to explore pain alleviators. According to a couple of doctors, I have an extraordinarily high pain tolerance. And how much pain I am willing to put up with in exchange for independence is absolutely my choice. I'm not making this decision today; I made this decision twenty years ago, and I thought about it for twenty years.

If I have to be in some pain in order to be coherent and present with my loved ones and to be as independent as possible, then I choose that. I have no doubt that you will all honor my intelligence and my integrity and my purpose. I am going to be independent as long as I am able. I will listen to everyone on my care team. And if we come to a point where there is a consensus that I should not do something, I will listen to that. I am strong-willed (I mean, you have met me), but I am not truculent. And if the pain is excruciating, I will definitely accept pain meds. I'm all for drugs for better living, as long as they are actually making me live better.

Treatment Options

Unless I see some overwhelming evidence that chemo, radiation, or surgery can extend the quality of my life as well as quantity, I will not submit to any of them. I have seen that journey at a horrifyingly close distance. Again, I made this decision twenty years ago. If I reach a vegetative/comatose state, don't put me on an IV. What is the point? To drag out being in a vegetative state??? Hell to the no!!!

How I Wish to Handle My Eventual Transition

I really hope I have a year or two before I have to worry about this, but just so you know my thinking, I don't want to spend any more time in a hospital than necessary. And I sure as fire do not want to die in a hospital or hospice institution.

Maranda has been so wonderful and gracious in giving me the freedom to die in her house. She also welcomes any of my friends and family to hang out, sleep over, whatever, here. I am so very grateful for this space. It is really rather ideal for such a situation.

When I get to the point where I am bedridden, I'd like to move my bed out into the larger basement area and arrange chairs and couches in such a way that lots of people can hang out at the same time. My only concern about doing that is the bathroom being further away from my bed. I might end up just moving all the furniture except the bed out of the bedroom and then moving some couches or futons in here in their place so that more people can hang out as comfortably as possible.

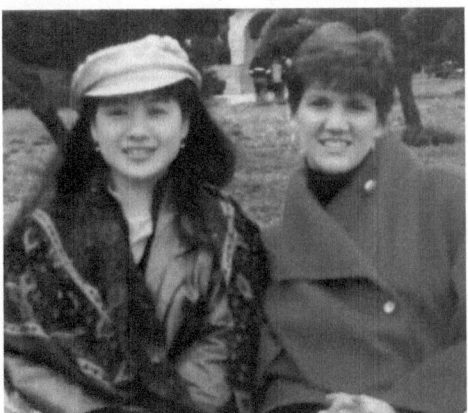

Hiroko and Me in Chicago 1993

When we get to my final one to two weeks of life (I know this is hard to gauge) I want Hiroko Kawamura to come from Japan and be my primary caregiver. She wishes the same. I want everyone else to be involved too, but Hiroko has a particular tenderness and a particular intimacy with my soul that I am really going to want at that time.

I used to dream about all my friends meeting each other at a wedding. A funeral or deathbed might also serve.

— · —

PART III: DUST IN THE WIND

(I MEAN, I AM FROM KANSAS)

23

— • —

WHY ME?

Do you consider yourself a philosophical person? If so, I bet you have encountered some real suffering in your life. I'd love to see some research about how many people with really sucky childhoods grew up to be philosophers. My gut instinct is probably a whole lot.

And if you're one of those people who feel like you don't have a philosophical bone in your body, you probably found yourself suddenly very contemplative indeed when you got your diagnosis and your own blind date with Grim.

I will warn you that this chapter is very philosophical. If you do not find enough agony here, please reread chapters Six through Fifteen, where I believe you will find more than enough agony for one lifetime. I do know the general terrain of your pain, dear readers. It's just that I experienced so much of it before my own diagnosis and got it healed that by the time I got there, I was very peaceful about it.

Why Is Not a Useful Question

June 13, 2020

So, for those of you who did not grow up in the Valley (No, I don't mean San Fernando or Silicon; I am referring to the one cozily situated in the Shadow of Death), getting your diagnosis probably made you break out in interrogatory seizures. These typically take the form of shaking your fists at the sky and screaming *Why* till your vocal cords are ragged with rage.

I wonder how culturally specific this impulse to demand a reason is. I think maybe all Americans have a *Why* chromosome, regardless of gender. When I lived in Korea, I once asked some Korean teachers and principals what was the most irritating thing about working with Americans. They said it was that we always have to know *why*. We can't just accept an order or an instruction. We must know the reason for it before we can move forward. And if we do not get a reason or we are not satisfied with the reason, we may opt not to cooperate.

The demand to know *why* comes at least partly out of the human rage for order. We feel we need to place our suffering in some framework where its placement makes sense to us, so we can see where it came from and where it's going, we can see how it relates to everything else in our life and the cosmos.

Of course, atheists will want to keep in mind that the question assumes an external locus of control, that something godlike outside of yourself is calling the shots and has singled you out for pain and has some purpose in doing so.

Most people who have a traditional view of God do not believe that evil comes from God, and yet God is the one to whom they direct their fury when circumstances beyond their own control befall them. Presumably, this is because even if God didn't send the pain, God didn't protect them from it, either. God let it happen.

I think it's at least moderately amusing that we rarely ask this question when good things happen to us. I have never heard of a single rich or beautiful person brooding over why they are rich or beautiful. If they were not born rich, they so often assume they made themselves rich by their own shrewd choices and somehow beautiful people often seem to unconsciously assume personal responsibility for their good looks, too.

But if they lose their fortune or are disfigured, they are way more likely to shake their fists at God and ask *Why*. So, if it's good, you did that yourself and are to be highly admired, but if it's bad, it's God's fault and S/he has deeply wronged you.

In *Night*, Elie Wiesel, holocaust survivor, answers the furious human accusation, "Where was God?" with a better question, "Where was man?" Ultimately, it is our responsibility to make sure that love conquers evil in this world. Back to rejecting that external locus of control. At such times, we may need to remind ourselves, "You are not a puppet being manipulated by some celestial Puppet Master above. You are already a 'real boy,' Pinocchio. Stop telling lies to yourself about your powerlessness."

You are animated by something that comes from inside, not outside. Either you want dominion over the earth or you don't. If you do, I feel like we should stop blaming God for everything undesirable that befalls us. It feels super why-ny. We need to focus on our own agency.

My Own Personal Why-ny Period

My own personal why-ny why-me period struck when I was in college. I looked at the life of my lovely friend, Soncee, and I looked at mine. Soncee was beautiful, kind, brilliant, charming, popular (still is). She was Miss Missouri and second runner-up to Miss America in 1990. Her parents were so loving and generous. Her brother was handsome and brilliant and kind. They seemed so rich to me.

Everything about her life seemed so ideal. She didn't have death and disability and poverty and stigma smeared all over her. She wasn't crippled by pain and trauma. I wanted God to explain to me what I did to deserve my life. I was a good girl, too. Why didn't I get a childhood and a family and a level of prosperity like that?

For years, I mourned for what I regarded as my lost childhood. I felt that God had dealt me a really rotten hand. Of course, it took growth and experience to come to realize that, 1) Soncee's life was probably not quite so idyllic as I imagined; 2) lots of people have suffered as much or more than me, and; 3) everything that happened to me helped make me more beautiful and interesting and strong than I would have otherwise been. Like a diamond or a star, the darker my background, the brighter I shine.

I believe I learned this from my own biography, but my friend Ashley, whose biography is infinitely more dramatic than mine, really articulated it well when she said, "*Why* is simply not a useful question."

The other thing I believe about the question is that once you have settled it in your mind, you don't need to return to it every time something else undesirable happens to you. So, by the time I got my own terminal cancer diagnosis, I didn't need to ask the question. I didn't shake my fist at God or rage.

I did direct a very strong "Really?!" in Her direction. "This is not how I would have written this story, but since you are a pretty powerful co-author,[1] I accept it. Let us proceed with the business at hand. If this is my last chapter, let me make it beautiful." The business at hand included some hard-core grief, but I had already answered my why questions to my satisfaction years prior. I could only do this because of the gut-wrenching experiences that preceded my own cancer.

Allow me to share with you some of what I concluded for myself in regard to the question *Why.*

Why Why? (Y^2)

It strikes me that we want to know why because not knowing leaves us with uncertainty and we humans are deeply allergic to uncertainty. When we are asking *why* in regard to the problem of pain, we want to know what caused it, where it falls in the long chain of cause and effect in our lives. I believe this effort to understand the cause or the reason for something is part of our effort to maintain some control, or at least the illusion of control.

If you want to read an eloquent spiritual answer to this question of why bad things happen to good people, you might be tempted to go all the way back to the book of *Job*, which is believed to have been written long before *Genesis*, though *Job*, like Solomon (or whoever was ghostwriting in his name) in *Ecclesiastes*, is more likely to make you want to stab yourself in the eye than provide you with a satisfactory answer. I mean, in the most cynical terms, the God of Job basically says, "Suck it up, I'm smarter than you. Oh, and here's a new family."[2] Let's just say that comforting is not their gift (nor apparently the purpose of those books) and leave it at that.

If you need companions in your grief, I recommend Pema Chödrön's *When Things Fall Apart*[3] (Buddhist) or Annie Dillard's *Holy the Firm*[4] or *For the Time Being*,[5] (Presbyterian/Catholic) which are beautiful and you may find them nourishing. Also, Harold Kushner's *Why Bad Things Happen to Good People*,[6] (Jewish), Philip Yancey's *Where Is God When It Hurts*[7]? (Evangelical), or *The Secrets of Divine Love* by A. Helwa[8] (Islamic).

In many faiths and many of these works, a common conclusion is that suffering both draws us nearer to God and makes us more like God. It brings out our divinity. It carves out beautiful reliefs in the walls of our souls. And Rumi (a Sufi Muslim), of course, says our wounds are how the light gets in.[9]

I happen to think that's true—that suffering can refine us—but just because it produces something meaningful doesn't mean that was its original purpose.

Cyanide is a naturally occurring substance that can kill you. But does that mean its *purpose* is to kill? Or is death simply one of its effects?

Likewise, if you subscribe to one of the Abrahamic faiths (Judaism, Christianity, Islam), you might believe that cancer is making you more like God. And if it shortens your life, maybe that purified spirit continues its journey in the next world. There *can* be purpose in suffering—but that doesn't necessarily mean suffering was *designed* for that purpose.

For a long time, that's how I coped with my own suffering. I chose to believe it could shape me into someone stronger, softer, more beautiful. That it could grow compassion, deepen empathy, stretch my capacity for generosity.

Since I'd already endured so much, I figured I might as well "embrace the suck," as the Marines say, and see if it could make me more awake, maybe even more spiritual. I wanted to believe my suffering could refine me, not just wound me. That it could purify something in me, not erase the pain, but make meaning from it.

As far as why goes, even if we don't wax philosophical and shake our fists at the sky demanding a spiritual reason for our cancer, we do usually at least want to know what the scientific explanation is for how our particular cancer came to be. Was it genetics? Red meat? Microwaves? Diet Coke? Air pods? Hair dye? What did I do????

In some cases, we might be looking for a culprit to blame, but in most cases I think it is just a natural human impulse to try to identify what entities or behaviors culminated in a deadly condition. If we survive, we can be sure to avoid that in the future and be better able to control whether we live or die. If not, at least our loved ones could avoid it. Knowledge is power. Knowing more can help us control more. That's one of the whys.

This desire to be in control is, of course, a manifestation of our intense resistance to uncertainty. Friedrich Nietzsche said so beautifully in 1889, "He who has a *why* to live can bear most any *how*."[10] This *why*, however, is not about what physical or spiritual forces caused our suffering, but the more important why: why do we go on? What propels us forward? What is the point of our lives?

And that brings me to a beautiful insight from Viktor Frankl (who may have just been channeling Buddha) in [Wo]Man's Search for Meaning: "Everything can be taken from a [person] but one thing: the last of the human freedoms—to choose one's attitude in any given set of circumstances, to choose one's own way."[11]

You don't get to choose every element of your narrative. Some ingredients life throws at you, and it is up to you to make something tasty out of them. You get to make your own recipe. Perhaps we feel that being able to see our suffering clearly and pinpoint it somewhere in logical space is the first step to formulating a response, the one thing we can control.

Now that I already have cancer, understanding how I got it is a bit of a moot point. I can no longer control that aspect of this situation. I can control how I decide to respond to cancer, whether I'm going to fight it, and how.

I cannot necessarily control whether I survive cancer. But if I do not survive, I do have some control over how I die.

My friend Stacy, who was an oncology nurse for years, laughed heartily when I informed her that I wanted to die elegantly. "Don't we all," she replied with a loving but skeptical chuckle.

You Can Make Your Own Meaning (D-I-whY)

The other point that Frankl makes is that human beings are meaning-making machines and you (and only you) get to decide what meaning to ascribe to any particular element of your biography. You choose your own why. That is the glory of being human.

If the quest to know why is really a quest for meaning, then maybe it is a useful question after all. But you don't have to be a "person of faith" to find meaning in the events of your life. You can ascribe to any event the meaning that you choose.

Here I can't help thinking of the movie *Airplane*, where the one guy says, "Johnny, what do you make of this?" handing him a newspaper. The other guy folds it up and puts it on his head, "A hat? A broach? A pterodactyl?"[12] His response may have been farcical, but you have to admire him for thinking outside the box. When life hands you a trash sandwich, you can do the same thing (make something creative out of it).

I love to find discarded things at garage sales, Goodwill, the side of the road, cart them home and restore them and redeem them, turn trash into treasure. I try to do the same thing with the events of my life. What do you make of this, Elisa? *I can make a hat, a broach...* I can make crap into something beautiful and creative.

I try to see everything that happens to me as the raw material out of which I may create a work of art. I see no point in wasting time complaining that I did not get better materials. I have been there and done that.

No amount of complaining is going to get Matilda-God to reshuffle the deck and deal me a new hand (if, in fact, she does all the shuffling herself). This is my culinary throw-down, and the clock is ticking. What delicious creation can I make out of this?

I have long contemplated getting a tattoo that says, *Every iota of my life redeemed*, which has been kind of a secret spiritual rallying cry for me for years. I mean that I want every moment, every experience I've ever had, whether it seemed good or evil, to be converted into something valuable, to be a seed that grows into a beautiful flower.

I want every drop of suffering along with every joyful experience to accrue to something I can use to feed the souls of others and my own, to bring more beauty into the world. I love that quote attributed to Abraham Lincoln, "I want it said of me by those who knew me best, that I always plucked a thistle and planted a flower where I thought a flower would grow."[13] And when those things in my biography that seem unredeemable cannot be made a seed, at least let them be fertilizer.

[Wo]man's Search for Meaning

Why is a question asked by thinking people, and yes, I realize that, especially with the ever-advancing prevalence of AI, they may constitute a small sample of the population. Many people rely on group-think and float along on platitudes they have absorbed through cultural osmosis. Those are the people who are most likely to blurt out brilliantly comforting lines like, *Everything happens for a reason.* And every time they do, you may be tempted to punch them in the throat.

I think that's because it does assume that external locus of control, the idea that someone or something outside of you is calling the shots. When people ejaculate this platitude, it's really hard not to feel they are trying to justify whatever you are suffering. That puts them squarely in the camp of Job's comforters, basically telling you that this is either good for you or you deserve it, and if so, then your agony is misplaced or illegitimate.

Everything happens for a reason feels perilously close to *Suck it up, Buttercup.* Is it any wonder that it makes us flinch? Such condolences are the verbal equivalent of wolves in sheep's clothing. They don't comfort; they intensify the pain.

But what if you were to reclaim this sentiment—and clarify that "everything happens for a reason" means *you* get to make up your own damned reason? That you can assign meaning to everything that happens to you. You—and only you—have the power to determine the significance of any part of your story.

Maybe it's more accurate to say: everything that happens to me has meaning because *I* assign that meaning. So instead of saying, "Everything happens for a reason," maybe try this: "Everything has meaning. And I'm the one who gets to decide what that meaning is."

So here I am with the trash sandwich of stage four pancreatic cancer before me and I am asking myself, "Elisa, what can you make of this?" I could rage about the injustice and pout and whine and be miserable, but I have already spent many years of my life drowning in agony. I'll be damned if I am going to waste any of this precious life I have left doing that.

And if your *why* is the *why bother, why go on* variety, I'm thinking if you have three months left to live, you could spend the whole time being miserable and complaining that you don't have more. You could waste all the life you have left, bemoaning the fact that this is all you get. It would be like having a little Chanel left in a bottle or a little Patron, and saying, "Because I don't have a whole bottle, I'm just going to cruise over here to the sink and pour this down the drain." Whoa! Or... and hear me out... you could decide to savor every last drop.[14]

Staying alive, keeping your body functioning and animated with that electric current we call life, is mechanical. But what is the purpose of being alive? I imagine most of us could agree that the mechanics of being alive only have value if we have some purpose, some reason for staying alive. Some appreciation for the life we are living.

So, I guess I think *why* is not useful if you mean, *Why did this happen to me?* However, the *why* that matters, the one that Nietzsche wrote about, *Why am I here?* That one matters more than anything. And no one can answer that for you but you.

No, this is not the fairy tale I would have written for myself, but I still don't have to let it turn into a horror story. If I only have a few months left to live, I am not going to spend those months being angry or focusing on the mechanics of trying to stay alive (more surgeries, more drugs, etc.) if that means I can't spend my days living my life meaningfully, loving people, leaving them with beautiful memories.

And we do not need *Why* for this, Beloveds.
We only need *What*.
And then *How*.

---

1. I still don't claim to know God's role in the painful situations in our lives, but I suppose she is a co-author in the extent to which she doesn't always prevent them.

2. A more reverent summation would be, you just can't understand the complexities of divine justice.

3. Chödrön, Pema. *When Things Fall Apart: Heart Advice for Difficult Times.* Shambhala Publications, 1997.

4. Dillard, Annie. *Holy the Firm.* Harper & Row, 1977.

5. Dillard, Annie. *For the Time Being.* 1st trade ed., Knopf, 1999.

6. Kushner, Harold S. *When Bad Things Happen to Good People.* Schocken Books, 1981.

7. Yancey, Philip. *Where Is God When It Hurts?* Zondervan, 1977.

8. Helwa, A. *Secrets of Divine Love: A Spiritual Journey into the Heart of Islam.* Penguin Random House India Private Limited, 2021.

9. Rumi. *The Essential Rumi.* Translated by Coleman Barks, HarperOne, 1995.

10. This is often attributed to Viktor Frankl but Nietzsche said it first and Frankl popularized it.

11. Frankl, Viktor E. *Man's Search for Meaning.* Translated by Ilse Lasch, Beacon Press, 2006.

12. Airplane! Directed by Jim Abrahams, David Zucker, and Jerry Zucker, performances by Robert Hays, Julie Hagerty, and Stephen Stucker, Paramount Pictures, 1980.

13. Humes, James C., editor. *The Wit and Wisdom of Abraham Lincoln.* Gramercy Books, 1996.

14. I know this seems obvious to many of us, but I have seen people giving up and at this stage in my cancer journey I was very conscious of the choice.

24

—·—

WHY I AM NOT AFRAID TO DIE

D o you let yourself think about whether you are afraid to die or do you just try to avoid bringing the subject up with yourself?

Death started punching me in the face before I even started kindergarten, so the question was hard to avoid. I got better at avoiding it as the years passed, but in my experience, Death is a stalker, and he would pop up terrifyingly at unexpected but pretty periodic times throughout my life.

Eventually, I got used to him and became less afraid.

What Does a 99-Year-Old Think When She Wakes Up Every Morning?

When I was forty-eight and forty-nine, the number fifty also haunted me like a scythe-bearing specter. I could see it peeking out from behind a corner just ahead—not far enough ahead for my taste. I couldn't even say the number aloud, much less look it straight in the eye.

Fifty seemed like the door to the other side of youth and once I passed through it, well, it seemed that then I would officially be on the road to death. I strongly suspected I was afraid of death. I was afraid of aging. I was afraid of facing the fact that my life would end at some point.

I guess that's why so many people hate birthdays. It's a reminder that the clock goes on ticking, whittling down your lifeline with each one-second tap. I remember years before when a friend had turned fifty and her elderly father just kept saying, "Half a pencil. Fifty is half a pencil." I guess, particularly if you are thinking about writing your life, that makes perfect sense.

All my life I have wondered how it feels to face your own death. I wondered about people who are over seventy, eighty, ninety—do they fear death? Does it loom over them? Is it any harder to put out of their minds than it was when they were younger? I always want to ask them, but I am also afraid to make them think about their own mortality (just in case it has not occurred to them).

I always wonder, *Does Betty White* [God bless her. At the time of this writing, she was still with us. May she rest in everlasting joy] *wake up and think, Today might be my last?* Is she afraid? Or is she just tired? I wonder if someone who is over ninety or one hundred is just tired and ready to rest.

There Are Fates Worse Than Death

Like I said, some people expressed surprise about how calm I have been in the face of death. To be honest, I was quite surprised myself. I always wondered if I would feel afraid. Much to my own amazement, it turns out I am not afraid to die.

Now, I'm not saying I relish the prospect. And I don't want to die suddenly. I quite prefer being able to take the time to say goodbye, arrange my own funeral, decide what lucky woman is going to get my fabulous shoe collection, make a disturbing video where I give my own eulogy... but now that I have a general idea that my expiration date is imminent and can plan accordingly, I feel peaceful about this.

The next thing you must understand... I don't know how to prepare you for this sentence, so I'm just going to hit you with it—

Death is not the worst thing that could happen to you.

In my case, the worst thing that could ever happen to me happened when I was four years old. It was the death of my three-year-old baby brother and my involvement in that event. An experience like that does provide one with a certain sense of sangfroid in the face of lesser losses. It also blows up your psyche like a car bomb, and the trauma fragments your brain into millions of tiny shards. It takes a very long time to put the pieces together again, and all the king's horses and all the king's men cannot do it for you.

I had so much help, and I am unspeakably grateful to all the people who have loved me and helped me find healing. You need lots and lots of help from lots of people to do this, but ultimately, you are the only person who can re-assemble your life. It took me almost fifty years to do so. But now that I know how, I can do it way faster. Which is handy since cancer just blew it up again.

For me, being responsible for someone else's death is the worst thing that could happen to you. Watching someone you love die in agony is the second worst. Abandonment is a close third. Your own death is possibly fourth.

That's just not the worst thing that could happen to you. It will suck a lot more for everyone you left behind than it will for you.

In Deborah Tannen's memoir, *Finding My Father*, she shares something her father told her over pizza one day when he was in his nineties that I just love. "I expect one morning to wake up and find myself dead, and I wouldn't mind. I wasn't alive before I was born, and I didn't mind at all."[1]

Being dead does not hurt. Anne Lamott likes to think of it as a "significant change of address."[2] I like that, too.

Entitlement Runs Deep

Another factor in my philosophy about my own demise was the realization that I had already lived longer than many people do. Just over a hundred years ago, the global average life expectancy was around thirty—largely because of high rates of infant and child mortality. Those who made it to adulthood often lived much longer, but I think people lived with a greater awareness of their mortality.

It is funny, in a really non-humorous way, how deep entitlement goes when you live in a wealthy nation in modern times with great medical care and a fairly long life expectancy. People seem to feel that they are entitled to live at least seventy years. And if they don't get to, they feel ripped off; they rage about the "injustice."

We are not born with a lifetime guarantee. None of us is actually entitled to seventy years... or even seven. Look at my dear Diane, who just got thirty. Or my sweet baby brother who only got three. I imagine that experiencing and witnessing their deaths is largely why I have always been keenly aware of the value and the beauty of life.

Yes, I kind of thought I'd live to be over a hundred and was planning accordingly. But I don't think I ever felt entitled to it. I think I was just always very conscious of the fact that any of our numbers could be up at any time.

Even before cancer, I loved this admonition from Arianna Huffington, *"Stop just assuming you have a full lifetime to do whatever it is you dream of doing."*[3] Life is happening now. In just the last couple of years, I have become so full of joy. Every breath of life is filled with such a sweet fragrance. I'm enjoying *now*.

Perhaps I Have Always Known I Was Living on Borrowed Time

I was, after all, just inches in front of my brother when he was killed. I survived. That has a profound impact on the psyche in so many ways. I know that I am not entitled to any amount of life. My focus has not been, *Why don't I get to live longer,* but *Why did I get to live this long?* I am so grateful for the years I have been given. And I have also achieved so much healing and happiness that I'm afraid most people never do.

All that joy and emotional wholeness provided me with resilience. I am happy with the life I have lived. I fulfilled my main mission. There are plenty of failures and unrealized dreams in my life, but I set out to live my life loving people, and I feel that I have been faithful to that mission since my childhood. I think perhaps this is another existential riddle: Am I satisfied with the life I have lived?

Eckhart Tolle reminds us that all we ever have is now.[4] And if I have fewer moments ahead of me than previously assumed, I'm sure the hell not going to spend them being miserable. I'm going to suck the nectar out of every moment, for my own sake, but I also want my loved ones to do that with the moments we have left to share. I want to be enjoyable so my loved ones can enjoy what they have left of me.

I also want to love those I love with what life I have left by preparing them for grief. I know that path intimately. I want to draw them a map before I go. I want to show them they can do this joyfully. Or at least, they can do it beautifully, without falling apart.

My life is full of love. I am surrounded by love, and my friends are absolutely amazing. They have made everything as easy and enjoyable for me as they could.

Hey Death, WTF??? What About My Effin' Best Laid Plans???
Tuesday, May 26, 2020

Yes, shortly after my diagnosis I wanted to scream, *Hey Death? Where the &%$# were you when I wanted to die all those years??* Where were you then, Hm??? I just want to shake you senseless—what is the MATTER with you??? I do not approve of your random ass ways!!!

Deep breath.

I don't know statistically how many people make it to 53. And I wouldn't want to be on the wrong side of that statistic.

Here's what I do know: I don't meet many people who seem as deeply content as I feel right now. And that's not a brag—it's a miracle. Somehow, against all odds, I've landed in this quiet, luminous place—in my mind, my heart, my relationships, my life. It feels almost like a kind of heaven.

I have so many streams of love flowing in and out of my days. I wish I knew more people who had discovered this kind of peace, this paradise that rises not from circumstances, but from the inside out.

For the record, I am highly unamused by Death's behavior.

But oh my God, Life!!! What did I ever do to deserve you??? You are so breathtakingly beautiful!!! You are so full of light and color and music and texture and fragrance!! You are hot and warm and cold and cool. You are wet and dry and hard and soft. Scratchy and silky and scaly and fury and feathery. You swim, you fly, you walk, you slither, you run, you lope, you burrow, you slide, you lie naked in the sun. You surprise me at every twist and turn.

And oh yeah, you, Death. Mortality, by any other name, you would still stink to high heaven. But, um, it's probably, maybe true that without you we would never be able to, um, taste life. We wouldn't even know what life was. We'd be like David Foster Wallace's fish being asked, *How's the water?* Turning to each other all mystified, *What the hell is water?*[5]

Do I have to thank you now? And can you make me mean it?? <Narrows eyes, shakes fist defiantly> Ugh. I might have to actually mean it.

But anyway... Let's talk about life!! bla blabla blabla blabla blabla...

I Have Looked Death Straight in the Eye

June 5, 2020

I (pompously?) posted this on Facebook about ten years ago, I think. Today I stand by it. I reserve the right to discover that I am wrong. That I have not looked my OWN death square in the eye, but I don't think so. I am not afraid now and I don't believe I'm going to be afraid.

I have walked through
the valley of the shadow of death

more than once and
I have looked death straight in the eye
and I can tell you this:

It is no match for the Divine Spirit
and the River of Life and Light
that flow through me!

Bring it, Grim!

I am NOT AFRAID OF YOU!!

You may slay me,
but by God, you cannot break me!
Live or die, I am not afraid of you!!!
For I have not been given a spirit of fear, but of
Love and of
Power and of
Sound Mind!

If I Worship You for Fear of Hell . . .

June 14, 2020

I just adore this prayer from the lovely, wise woman, Rabia al-Adawiyya al-Qaysiyya, a Sufi mystic from the 8th century:

Oh Lord, if I worship You
because of fear of hell,
then burn me in Hell;
if I worship You because I desire Paradise,
then exclude me from Paradise;
but if I worship You for Yourself alone,
then deny me not Your eternal beauty.[6]

There is such courage in this kind of love—so unbargained, so total. It is the kind of love I hope to offer in the presence of death: ungrasping, full-hearted, stripped of striving. Just love for love's sake.

1. Tannen, Deborah. *Finding My Father: His Century-Long Journey from World War I Warsaw and My Quest to Follow*. Ballantine Books, 2020.

2. Lamott, Anne. *Traveling Mercies: Some Thoughts on Faith*. Anchor Books, 2000.

3. Huffington, Arianna. *"Stop just assuming you have a full lifetime to do whatever it is you dream of doing."* Facebook, 16 June 2018.

4. Tolle, Eckhart. *The Power of Now: A Guide to Spiritual Enlightenment*. New World Library, 1999.

5. Wallace, David Foster. *This Is Water: Some Thoughts, Delivered on a Significant Occasion, About Living a Compassionate Life*. Little, Brown, 2009. Yes, I realize I've used this metaphor twice, once for trauma and once for life. It's just so perfect for both.

6. Rabia al-Adawiyya. *Early Sufi Women*. Translated by Rkia Elaroui Cornell, Fons Vitae, 1999, p. 115.

25

— · —

THE MUCH-MALIGNED SHADOW OF DEATH

I'm curious. Which do you avoid more assiduously? Snakes or the subject of death? (Or are you one of those weird Goth Slytherins, besties with both?) I imagine that our aversion to death is like most people's fear of snakes—really deeply encoded in our DNA, designed to improve our life expectancy. But given how much death is a part of life, it really does not serve us to run every time it raises its homely hoary head.

Why You Do Not Run from Suffering and Death
June 15, 2020

Talk about suffering here below... Well, there is a beautiful spiritual in a haunting minor key that begins with those words. Many of you will know the rest. Phil Keaggy has a lovely version.[1]

I have miles of Judeo-Christian scripture winding around the hallways in my brain, so forgive me if it is my first go-to source of language and literary allusion. The apostle Paul said a lot of weird and paradoxical things. One of them was, "I rejoice in my suffering."[2] I'm taking that a bit out of context, but in that single clause he is definitely saying that these two states are not mutually exclusive (he is also saying that suffering can be a cause for joy).

Those things that bring us joy and those things that cause us suffering are all sown together, like the weeds among the wheat. We do not alternate between happy and sorrowful, as if there were two pure states of being on either side... the streams of pain run throughout, along with streams of joy, one ebbing and the other flowing at each turn and with the passing of the seasons, and sometimes both ebbing or both flowing. But if we are awake and our eyes are open, neither stream ever dries up altogether.

It somehow took me decades to learn that pain and joy are not mutually exclusive. In fact, I think they are actually sort of symbiotic. I am deeply persuaded that the depth of pain you are able to feel is proportionate to the depth of joy you can feel—and that you learn to recognize, see, discern, appreciate joy precisely because you know its absence.

We usually fear pain and look around for the exit signs as soon as we get the faintest whiff of its acrid stench wafting towards us. We want an escape or a way around.

The Antidote Is IN the Venom

John Locke, the *Lost* cast member, not the philosopher (but presumably named after him), showed the younger character, Boon, a cocoon and explained how he could help its resident get free of the stuff that was binding him in, but if he did, that moth would not survive, because it is the struggle that forges strength.[3] If you cut the struggle, you cut the strength. No two ways about it.

And I guess I believe that your ability to feel joy depends on the strength you develop by learning how to walk through suffering and not keep looking for a way around it. You have to be strong to feel the joy, at the same time you are feeling anguish. That butterfly needs to be strong so she can experience the joy of soaring through the air, floating on the (notably all too uncertain) wind.

I believe there are planes we reach where we have become mature and have found a peace with much of the pain of both the past and the present. These are successive planes, stages we pass through, milestones we reach. Some of the peace is because we find healing and the pain diminishes.

But there will always be some pain as long as we are alive, and as long as we love—you can't love anyone and not know pain—either that which they cause (no matter how unintentionally), or that which you feel for them as they suffer in their own journeys, or as their journeys in this lifetime come to a close and you feel the deep pain of grief. You will never reach a stage in this life where you are free of pain, unless you anesthetize, and that is not life.

Don't be depressed or disheartened by this fact, Dear Ones. There is so much joy in all of this. The more life you live, the more suffering you see, the more joy you find. It is a great paradox, but true—if you run from suffering and death, you run from life, too.

You can't really taste how sweet life is when you don't know how precious it is. You don't know what beauty is unless you know what ugly is. You don't know what joy is unless you know what sorrow is. And too often you don't know you're alive until you've come face to face with the alternative.

It is a sacred, beautiful place to be. And when you know that you are loved more than anything in the world, by entities both human and divine, and that you are completely safe in that love, whether you live or die, you can find joy even in the darkest places. You can actually find and feel more joy precisely because of the darkest, most angst-filled places. Let us then join Paul in his weird wisdom and find a way to rejoice in our suffering.

And if you're not crazy about the way Paul talks about it, consider Maulana[4] Rumi's words in the Masnavi (as translated by Moezzi and Moezzi):

Don't retreat, come near.
Don't lose faith, adhere.
Seek the tonic nectar in the bitter sting.
Go to the source of the source of your spring.[5]

It's not just that there is healing on the other side of death. There is healing *in* the grief, *in* the death. The healing is hidden in the loss itself.

The Shadow of Death Is Not Black, It's Technicolor
June 2, 2020

Do not be afraid of the dark, my loves. Don't be afraid that the shadow of death from my accelerated biography is going to touch you and bring you darkness or snuff out your light. Shadows only exist where there is light! And this is a sacred space, my life, this chapter. The light of God is shining through the exquisite stained glass of my life... actually, you know that stained glass that is a mosaic of thick chunks of glass? It's like that!

There has been so much brokenness... but... the Spirit can put broken pieces together in a way that is even more beautiful than the original whole (I hasten to add this cannot be done without our enthusiastic collaboration). Each piece is stained with so many different kinds of experiences, both painful and ecstatic, an array of experiences that evoke emotions we don't even have names for.

She has done that with the broken shards of my life. I am very pleased with the work of art She has made of my heart. It calls me to worship. It calls me to love. It calls me to share my healing.

Her light filters through this strange prism of my life, and as a near miraculous result, these shadows of mine are alive! They flicker and dapple with motion. They are mixed with glorious light and all these mesmerizing, vibrant, dancing colors.

Trust me, you want some of that, friend! You want some of the holiness that flows and buzzes with mystery in the thin spaces between one realm and the next. It feels like magic, and I want to share it with you. Not because it's *mine*, but because it flows through me—from the divine—as it flows through you, too. I'm just learning how to notice it.

And if I can, I believe you can, too. I would that you, too, would suddenly see the world in technicolor 3-D, to be fully present in every single seemingly mundane moment, along with those that are more obviously precious, as this "acceleration" is enabling me to do. To find the miraculous in the mundane.

I remember a precious moment when my sweet Diane was recovering from one of her surgeries, when she could finally stand on her own again over the sink and wash her own hands. She was so delighted. The beauty and freedom in that very simple act—that moment never left me. I feel like I have never taken such things for granted since.

All week I have had this quote of Jesus speaking to Peter floating in the back of my mind: "Truly I tell you, when you were young, you dressed yourself and walked where you wanted to. But when you are old, you will stretch out your hands, and another will dress you, and carry you where you do not want to go."[6] I exult in the ability to stand up and go wherever I will and do whatever I wish, as long as I can.

And so, my friends, when you stand in the shower and feel warm water spilling over every inch of your thirsty skin, I urge you, be filled with amazement and joy as it sates you, as it cleanses you. Take joy in your own strength to stand up straight and bathe yourself. When you bend over the sink to brush the miracles of your teeth, think of the wonder that we have bodies that bend and twist and rotate in so many lovely ways. When you taste the toothpaste, aware of the privilege of tasting anything and acknowledge this tiny blessing that you can have an experience of pleasant taste while doing something that is simply practical and necessary—it is a chore, it does not have to have any aesthetic joy in it, and yet it does.

It feels good to have the bristles brush your teeth and gums, to find your "pearly whites" delightfully smooth when you are finished, to have the joyful sensation of fresh water in your mouth, to experience that taste of toothpaste or mouthwash that you have chosen to your preference. I could go through every moment of your day like this, but why deprive you of the pleasure of your own mindful appreciation of the beauty in each drop of your life?

My prayer is that the colorful shadows of my final chapter will spill joyfully over into whatever chapter you are writing now. I hope that in this way I might bring you more joy than sorrow if you follow my journey. I wish, my beloveds, that you could be as alive as I am now!

While Yet in Possession of the Extravagant Gift of Life

How sad would it be if I spent my days mourning while I am yet in possession of this great extravagant gift of life? If I go on as I have been, and I wish to, I will have days full of joy, as if joy were the canvas, punctuated here and there with moments of poignant grief as I prepare myself to lose each beautiful soul that I have come to adore.

Grief is beautiful, too—each sorrow a kind of exotic flower, painted with the same glory that allowed Georgia O'Keeffe to show us what we'd never truly seen.[7] Her gift was not just in painting flowers, but in *seeing* them—so fully, so intimately—that we couldn't help but see them differently, too.

Artists like O'Keeffe offer us their eyes. They remind us to linger. To notice. To stop letting beauty slip in one eye and out the other. Let us instead receive these images fully, let them enter both eyes and burn themselves onto the walls of our imagination, so we may carry them with us always.

This year I have been envisioning souls as beautiful flowers that are fed by the light that other souls shine on them through their love, through their loving gaze. You need the light of the divine to flourish. So often She pours that light into you through other souls who have opened themselves to being conduits of love. Please be one of those. And surround yourself with those.

Don't live your life in black and white, Sweet Ones. And do not make the mistake of thinking that the shadow of death is black, or monochrome, or sinister. I do not believe it is. There is light, there is color, and there is safety here. Perhaps you can see this shadow as a protective one and lean into the cry of David (as I am), "Keep me as the apple of your eye, hide me in the shadow of your wings." [8]

---

1. Keaggy, Phil. *Talk About Suffering*. Performance by Phil Keaggy, included on *Way Back Home*, Myrrh Records, 1986.

2. Romans 5:3.

3. *Lost*. Created by J.J. Abrams, Jeffrey Lieber, and Damon Lindelof, performance by Terry O'Quinn, season 1, episode 7, "The Moth," directed by Jack Bender, ABC, 3 Nov. 2004.

4. Maulana is a term of respect that means something like "our revered teacher."

5. Moezzi, Melody. *The Rumi Prescription: How an Ancient Mystic Poet Changed My Modern Manic Life*. TarcherPerigee (Penguin Group), 2020.

6. John 21:18.

7. Lisle, Laurie. *Portrait of an Artist: A Biography of Georgia O'Keeffe*. Washington Square Press, 1986.

8. Psalm 17:8.

LIFE IS NOT BEAUTIFUL BECAUSE IT IS LONG

Storing Treasures Where Moth and Rust Do Not Destroy

June 1, 2020

I am drawn to you like the
primeval moth to the flame.
In my heart, I know that the intensity
of these feelings of love cannot endure forever—

So while they are pouring forth
from so generous a spring,
let us drink from them, inhale them even,
until we are giddy and satiated,
that we may also feed upon the memories
as long as we each shall live.

(You keep savoring those moments on my behalf, as long as you each
shall live, my beloveds...)

Striving After Wind

When my friend Diane was dying, she continued to be meticulously obsessed about her dental hygiene. She had beautiful teeth, and I always helped her with them, but I wince to recall that I laughed once when she asked for help brushing them. It seemed so absurd to me when she had weeks left to live, she should give any care at all to something so (now) inconsequential as her teeth.

In a previous chapter, I spoke of the utter pointlessness of daily activities that I felt for a couple of days early in my diagnosis. I sympathized with Israel's golden king writing in his despondency (and it's worth noting, that guy had everything – hundreds of beautiful wives, more money than God, a Mensa worthy brain, all the power in the world – what did he have to be depressed about?!), "All is futility and striving after wind."

When You Live in the Moment

Wednesday, May 27, 2020

That first day I had come home and started putting my books away because I thought I would never need this brain again, so what was the point in investing in it? I have absolutely nothing to plan for now, no way to use any potential learning in the future. I wondered why one would use the treadmill when she had been given mere months to live. Doesn't matter how long my heart lasts, it and everything else will be long gone by the time it was supposed to have extended my life expectancy.

It seemed that the only worthwhile activities would be those that would have some long-term effect. I thought I should focus on writing love letters to my dearest ones.

But here's the thing (I know you were dying to find out where the thing was, and I am so pleased to be the one to locate it for you), and I know you are going to raise your eyebrows, but I love those activities! Yes, I even love the treadmill! I got on one day that first week saying, "I'm just going to go twenty minutes, lightly." But thirty-five minutes later I was trotting along having completely forgotten about my twenty-minute target. And I was feeling great!

Endorphins are an important reason to keep doing the treadmill. Also, my brain works really well on the treadmill—my right and left brain are busily passing notes back and forth, giving rise to creative new thoughts and revelations, seamlessly knitting them all together. The treadmill can be a very intellectual activity as well as a key to emotional health (besides the physical benefits).

And as for learning, oh my, I love to read and learn! I think my nerdiness is encoded in my DNA. Knowledge is delicious! Like chocolate, it doesn't have to be useful. It gives me joy! And if it gives me joy, that's a damned good reason to keep doing it. Many of these endeavors that we think of as being future oriented have so much intrinsic value right here in the present moment of doing them.

In doing these things, I am living in my brain and my body. I am enjoying my physical and intellectual existence. Maybe heaven, or one of them, is being right here in this moment, enjoying it. If you can't enjoy this present moment, what makes you think you can enjoy any moment?

I, for example, am sitting here on my bed typing away and my heart is full of joy. I love thinking and writing! I love knowing that people I love are going to enjoy what I write and maybe even be inspired by some of it. Maybe even changed, (dare I say the word out loud?!)

And let us recall those well-worn (because well-loved) words of Thoreau,

I went to the woods because I wished to live deliberately, to front only the essential facts of life, and see if I could not learn what it had to teach, and not, when I came to die, discover that I had not lived. I did not wish to live what was not life, living is so dear; nor did I wish to practice resignation, unless it was quite necessary. I wanted to live deep and suck out all the marrow of life, to live so sturdily and Spartan-like as to put to rout all that was not life, to cut a broad swath and shave close, to drive life into a corner, and reduce it to its lowest terms... [1]

The only way we ever truly live is by being present in the moment, savoring each drop of life, not busily, frantically cycling through moments as fast as we can to get to some future moment where, we think, we will really be happy. When you live in the moment, you find joy in what you are doing in the moment, and you pursue those things that bring you joy. Life is just a long string of potentially beautiful moments to be savored—or not.

Another Note on the Beauty of Life's Transience
Wednesday, May 27, 2020

Now, don't break out in hives because I am going to use the word "Jesus." I do not identify as an evangelical, though I was raised one, but I still find so much beauty in many parts of scripture.

Jesus said, "Don't even worry about tomorrow because tomorrow has enough worries of its own."[2] Ain't that for damned sure. And then he talks about the beauty of the Lilies of the Field, who do not toil or spin or in any way dress themselves. And yet the golden king himself was not dressed as gloriously as one of those flowers.

There's something so beautiful about the lack of permanence in life. The ancient Greeks celebrated it in their fantastic worlds of gods and humans. Humanity's gift is mortality. Everything we do has meaning and significance precisely because of our mortality—something the gods will never know nor enjoy.

There is joy and excitement in the uncertainty of the life of a mortal. It makes each moment so very beautiful, so very precious. Every moment reminds us, if we are mindful enough to lean in and take note, that we shall never pass this way again.

My life has just become a great illustration of this beauty of transience. Beloved friends, we must treasure each other and the opportunities that we have from time to time to walk into each other's hearts and enjoy the wild beauty there, the flowers of wisdom sculpted in such fragile organic bodies, the tender affection that has sprung up as lovely as the flowers of the field. Let us breathe in the fragrance of those flowers, which are here today and gone tomorrow, and allow it to be imprinted on the memories of our souls.

When the Diagnosis Is Grave
Wednesday, August 5, 2020

Dear Ones, I wrote this about five years ago when a friend's mother had been diagnosed with pancreatic cancer. God knows I have had my share of grief, and you probably will, too, if you have not already. We all have our Trail of Tears to traverse, but some of those are tears of joy. Life is a complicated cocktail of agony and ecstasy. You will never fully know the latter, Dears, save you drink the whole cup to its dregs.

When the diagnosis is grave, you turn away from that ugly pun that is trying to push itself in your face. Graves are the last thing you want to think about right now and you can see this one barreling towards you like a boulder let loose from a mountain crag, tearing down the mountainside to the highway you've been blithely driving along.

When you close your eyes, you can see the spinning, rolling gravestone getting ever nearer. You open them to drive the apparition away. You look for bright things around you to anchor your soul to this moment. You cannot lose this precious moment, cannot let it be lost in thinking about what is to come.

Do not skip ahead, Loves. However soon or late that tombstone arrives, you can't waste one single instant of time between now and then. You cannot let any life be poured out in the dirt and wasted as if there were any excess, as if life were so abundant and so cheap that there could be some bit you considered waste and threw away.

That tombstone may be the capstone of a beautiful life... the reminder that our days are precious precisely because of their paucity. Grief is the price of love, they say. Do not forget that the ecstasy is right there mixed with the agony. You must drink the one to have the other. It's a fair trade.

The adoring woman who poured out $20,000 of pure nard on Jesus' feet "to prepare him for burial" understood this, washing his feet with her tears and filling the room with the fragrance of love-infused gratitude and grief.[3] When the diagnosis is grave, you probably will be crushed by that cold, ominous tombstone.

Suffer yourself to be crushed like an olive, for the crushing is the only way to release its essence, that mysterious healing oil produced by brokenness. Each drop of life is a priceless gift! Each drop of grief is priceless, too. Each drop of healing nascent within you more precious than thousands of dollars' of nard. Break the vial. Release the healing. Consume them all, My Loves, that after the crushing, you may be made fully whole and reach this consummation of your souls.

Life Is Not Beautiful Because It Is Long

Monday, June 1, 2020

It is beautiful because it is deep and filled with joy, filled with love, filled with grace, filled with wonder. Due to several early experiences, I have never taken life for granted, but particularly after I watched my beloved Diane die at the tender age of thirty, I have been keenly aware of the value and the beauty of life, though for too many of the last twenty years I was in too much existential pain to truly savor it.

In just the last couple of years, I have become so full of joy. Every breath of life is filled with such a sweet fragrance. For some reason peonies are my favorite floral fragrance, and their season is very brief. Whenever I pass them, I try to stop, bury my nose in their fluffy petals, and breathe deeply, inhaling their fragrance into my soul. I like to think that the fragrance of life is like that. It is sweet, and very transient.

I have a dear student whose Zoom picture only comes up in black and white. We tease her about being trapped in the 1950s. Since May 22, I feel the opposite. My life is being broadcast in brilliant technicolor, 3D... everything is so sharp and clear and lovely. I try to feel everything, every sensation, every emotion. There is joy underlying everything. Grieving joyfully does not mean there is no pain or other emotions; it means that joy is your default state.

I got mad at the tech one day early in my cancer sojourn because he insisted I had to have a pregnancy test before my CT. I gave him a litany of very convincing reasons why this was unnecessary, each of which I thought sufficient in itself. I never (rarely?) get mad at strangers and my "mad" was very mild. It consisted of me telling him vehemently through the muffles of my mask that I was deeply offended. I all but stomped upstairs to the lab to check in, huffing and puffing and fuming.

Then he came up, and we realized that we both thought it was already June and had miscalculated the dates of my last period. How we both did that, I don't know. But when he realized it, I was saved the humiliation. My soul was still ringing with all the emotion though.

When I left the hospital, noticing every step I took down the staircase, very mindful and present in each footfall, I thought, *There is joy even in fury. There is joy in being able to feel anything. There is joy in having a full range of emotions to experience while you are yet alive.*

And in addition to being technicolor 3-D, my life has been turbocharged this week. So much to do, no idea how much time left to do it. So much to feel, to experience, to express, to achieve. I end every day utterly exhausted, and I think it has more to do with how alive and alert I am than any actual changes in my body. Not 100 percent clear on that yet. I'm assuming what has changed most about my body is my awareness of it.

Anyway, people take lots of illicit drugs to get the feelings I'm having—to amplify their experiences, their feelings, the totality of their lives. And here I am getting it for free. Drug free, anyway. I'll count the other costs later.

I have had a mantra for five or six years that I can belt out with even more authenticity today than I have been for the last five: *I am full of light, full of love, full of joy, and full of God!*

Again, I hope you will not get your knickers in a knot that I used the word *God*. I think there is something bigger than me, bigger than all of us, something we all share, that connects us, that inspires us (you know *inspire* literally means *to put breath or infuse spirit into someone*, those seeds of creativity that float into our minds on some holy wind and come out as works of art). I am full of that.

And so are you. I love that quote that has been attributed to Einstein, who did not identify as a religious person: There are only two ways to live—as though nothing is a miracle, or as though everything is. I think Miracles are us. Miracles flow through us. Every atom and every moment is a miracle. You don't have to see it. You don't have to acknowledge it. There is so much more joy available to you when you do.

---

1. Thoreau, Henry David. *Walden; or, Life in the Woods.* Ticknor and Fields, 1854.

2. Matthew 6:34

3. John 12:1-8.

— • —

PART IV: TRAGEDY AND TRANSFORMATION

27

— · —

METAPHORS I LIVE BY

The Principle of Linguistic Relativity

Benjamin Lee Whorf was originally an insurance assessor who noticed that when an empty gasoline drum was so marked ("Empty Gasoline Drum") people were a lot more likely to blow themselves up by smoking in front of it than if it were marked "Gasoline drum."[1]

This led him to ponder the power of words to guide our thoughts in one direction or another. Whorf eventually became a linguist and formulated what is now known as the Whorfian hypothesis or the principle of linguistic relativity. In its strong form, it posits that we can't think a thought we don't have a word for.

Well, simple circumlocution proves that this is not exactly the case. We don't have the word *schadenfreude* in English, but we can certainly understand the concept of feeling glee at someone else's downfall or comeuppance when the word is explained to us and no doubt many have had no trouble having that thought even before they had a slick, zeitgeisty German word to express it with.

So, the weaker form (and I'd rather use a word like *tempered* than *weak*, thus partly illustrating my point) of the principle is that the words we have heavily influence the direction of our thought. If you think *this is a gasoline drum*, you are likely to focus on the flammable fumes part, whereas if you add the word *empty*, you may deemphasize the deadly nature of the drum in question and pulling out a cigarette, greatly hasten your own demise.

So, my question is, how do I talk about cancer so that it is not in the driver's seat? How do I talk about myself as a person who is contending with cancer? Am I a victim? A patient? A warrior? A survivor? A cancernaut? How do my words shape my attitude to my experience and thus affect my actions? Since I am a bona fide word nerd (aka, linguist), I thought very intentionally about the way words shape my experience of cancer.

I Do Not Wish for War Within

July 21, 2020

Don't we have a better metaphor for eliminating cancer? Aren't we sick of war yet? Sick to death of all the death, destruction, and devastation? Sick of considering everyone who is different from us as the enemy? Of steeling ourselves for a fight every time we find our wishes do not accord with those of the other?

I wonder if any one of us could go a whole day without using any language that is part of a war metaphor. Deborah Tannen has written a whole book about this called *The Argument Culture*.[2] War seems to be engraved on our hearts and written into our DNA. War is our go-to metaphor for dealing with opposition.

No wonder literal war is the first knee jerk reaction of most individuals and governments. We can scarcely conceive of countering opposition outside this metaphor. Our guiding metaphor for dealing with difference or opposition is violence.

As a linguist, I am deeply tuned into the idea that your words determine your thoughts (you can't do a lot of thinking without words. Some yes, but not a lot) and then, of course, your thoughts determine your actions. If you want to act right, to change your behavior, you should start with your words.

War is certainly the go-to metaphor for responding to cancer. And I don't like it. I don't want to be coerced into using a metaphor that contradicts my core values. I do not want to visualize anything killing something else inside my body, not even a tumor. I want them gone, but must I resort to violence to resolve them? I cannot promise you I will be able to eliminate them entirely from my speech or writing as I forge my way onward in this journey, but I think I shall try.

I think on reflection, I am ok using the warrior metaphor for the person who is in mortal combat with cancer, but not as a metaphor for what is going on inside my body. I like the idea of cancer warriors claiming their power, marshalling their strength, overcoming against poor odds.

Other Metaphors for Cancer Resolution
Tuesday, June 21, 2020

Isn't there some way we can reconceptualize the process of eliminating the cancer to something more in accordance with the way we think the world should work? I don't want to imagine little soldiers running through my veins, throwing grenades, getting blown up by IEDs.

I'm thinking of someone scaling an imposing mountain. Many people will turn that into a war metaphor, too: the mountain is the foe, and either you win, or she wins, but there can be only one winner. (Now don't mistake me, I do not want cancer to win anything).

However, in a situation like that, you have the option of considering the mountain to be a collaborator in your success. You are working with the mountain. (And if it were me, why would I climb a mountain I do not love? I want to love the mountain as I scale it). If I don't want to think of cancer as a collaborator, I can think of the cells in my body as collaborators.

And now I'm thinking about my baby brother at about three, not long before he died, trying to get the wrinkles out of the bedspread after we made the bed. He walked around the bed, pinching at each wrinkle as if he could remove them by lifting them out of the bedspread. I imagine the mystified look on his adorable little face trying to get his head around how an action over there at the side of the bed, pulling on the spread, could remove something from the middle. I'm not settling on this metaphor; I'm just exploring it. Making tumors disappear like wrinkles.

Ah! I know! I think I like the metaphor of washing! Love, in the form of chemo, washing cancer out of my body. Yes! I like that one best. To be washed and cleansed and "sanctified," to be made sacred again. To be cleansed of cancer. EPOCH-R might be a power washer, and more power to it. I wish to be washed.

<Starts singing I'm gonna wash that cancer right out of my hair [3] Well. I mean. Maybe my wig?> I see Love washing cancer right out of my body. Cleansing is a far more redemptive metaphor than killing.

Cancer to Society (Malignancy Maligned?)
Monday, October 19, 2020

On the other hand, cancer itself is used as a metaphor. "You are a cancer on society! You must be cut out!" It is possibly the most scathing recrimination in our metaphorical imagination. We spit this aspersion with a venom of the highest toxicity—it is so reprehensible that we often resort to calling it "the c word," as if the occlusion of five of its letters would dull this existential scalpel that threatens to slice through our death denying defenses.

Yet many have said that cancer is a gift, that it opened their eyes to life and helped them savor it—made them truly alive. Being introduced to death changes the way you see your life forever. Nobody knows how to celebrate life like those of us who have come face to face with its alternative.

Others mock them.

The mockers you will have always with you.

But cancer has another magical property. It is a magnet that reaches across the miles and decades and pulls hearts back to you. It resurrects old ties that seemed long severed. It pulls the broken pieces of discarded relationships back together and restores them to wholeness. At least it can. It did for me.

Where time and distance had reduced a relationship to a tiny little spark in the heart, cancer breathes upon those sparks like a benevolent fiery dragon (you know, of the lucky, Chinese variety) and reignites them. Paradoxically, the flames grow into beautiful conflagrations that warm you while you shiver in the icy grip of the disease.

Cancer also casts a lens over your eyes that not only shows the world in brilliant hues you had not noticed before, it casts a laser-like spotlight over every person in your life, bathing them in an appraising light.

You suddenly know exactly who is important to you, and you are able to let insubstantial connections fall away and be forgotten. I realized there were people from my past I was content to leave in the past. They only crossed my path for a season. Their work in my life is done, and mine in theirs. They may have been woven into my biography, but they had not been woven into the fabric of my soul. I did not tell them about my cancer.

But others... others dear to me with whom I had had no substantial contact for twenty, thirty, forty years, came flowing back like waves from a vast ocean of love that I didn't even know belonged to me. This truly amazed me. I did not know all those people loved me so much. The mockers you will have always with you, but you will not always have me. Your dearest loved ones... all have an expiration date. Cancer slaps you across the face and pulls you out of the trance that the repetitive rhythm of daily life has drawn you into. "Read my lips," it says. "This is not for play. Death is for keeps. And time is always running out."

So, what is cancer to society, really? It can be a beautiful agent of change in our individual lives and in our relationships. It can be a call to love. I am not venerating disease or fetishizing suffering, but catastrophe can always be a call to love. Anything can.

I am so delighted and humbled by all those who have answered that call.

Cancer is a CT for Your Soul

I've heard more than a few people scoff at the idea that cancer should have any positive effect on them. They say it didn't change them, and they deeply resent the expectation that they *should* be more grateful or somehow transformed after such an ordeal. And honestly? I get that. I cannot speak for everyone's cancer experience. Each diagnosis unfolds within its own unique biography—framed by what came before and what follows.

That said, I would offer two gentle questions—not as judgment, but as invitation to reflection. First: What kind of grief or adversity had you faced before cancer? If this was your first great reckoning, it may have landed in your life with a very different emotional architecture than mine did.

Second: What narratives, if any, lit the way for you? Did you have a story, a person, a philosophy, that helped you make sense of what was happening? The metaphors we inherit or create can be lifelines (or deadly anchors).

For me, it was Marcus Aurelius—though I didn't know his name at the time. I just held onto this sense that what stands in the way *becomes* the way.[4] That suffering could be meaningful, if I stayed awake for it. (I'll admit, if I had a child, I might have experienced cancer with far less equanimity. I hope not—but I'll never claim to know how someone else's thresholds might differ.)

I've come to see suffering as a kind of scalpel—or maybe a chisel. It can destroy, or it can shape something more beautiful than what was there before. It can cut or it can carve. A great deal, I believe, comes down to agency—to what you choose to do with what life has handed you. You alone have the power to change your inner state. (And my God, it takes time! It took me twenty years to change my inner state. I am in no way presenting agency as an instant panacea).

When they looked inside my body with a CT, they found something I didn't know was there. And in a strange way, cancer invited me to do the same—to look inside my soul. I didn't find diamonds or gold bars. But I did find buried treasure: strength I hadn't tested, courage I didn't know I owned, peace where I expected panic.

If we had a CT scan for the soul, what might it show? Untapped gifts? Starving hopes? Unfinished grief? You've been busy living. Maybe you forgot to open some of those inner gifts. Maybe you didn't even know they were there. But this experience, however brutal, might be the thing that draws your attention back inward.

In my case, Diane's death was my first spiritual CT. It revealed tumors of unresolved grief. Years later, when my own cancer diagnosis came, it was my second spiritual CT and it showed me that I had done the inner healing, and the scan was surprisingly clear. I wasn't afraid to die. I was calm. Not because I'm heroic, but because I'd done the work.

Your scan may show you something else. You may discover that you haven't been feeding your soul, and that you're spiritually undernourished. If so, cancer may be the wake-up call that saves your life, even as it threatens it. It may help you find your purpose, recover your joy, or uncover a deep well of resilience.

Or—it may not. That's okay too. You are the one who gets to decide what it all means. That's not toxic positivity. That's sacred agency.

I Shall Not Reduce Myself to the Identity of Cancer Patient

One of the most important ways to take away cancer's keys is to limit and control the centrality of cancer to your identity. You build your own identity through language, both the way you talk about yourself and the way you talk to others.

I decided that one of the best ways to reclaim my identity—and resist being reduced to my cancer diagnosis—was to stop referring to myself exclusively as a cancer patient and to gently push back when others did. I even tried to make this point (with a wink) in one of the many titles I toyed with for this book: *Stage Four Cancer ((Not All That)) Patient.* Yes, I thought it was clever too. Literally, the word *patient* means "one who suffers." And sure, that's appropriate on several levels, but I didn't want it to be the only story told about me.

In grammar and linguistics, the *patient* of a sentence is essentially the direct object—the one being acted upon. In *She kissed a frog*, the frog is the patient, acted upon by the princess (though who suffers most in that scenario is debatable—I've always thought I'd rather just keep the talking frog).

Some people prefer to see themselves as cancer warriors. Others reject the martial metaphor but also find it a bit tedious to keep saying *the person who has cancer*. Many choose the term cancer survivor, sometimes even before survival is assured, as a way of promoting a self-fulfilling prophecy. Personally, I've never felt entirely comfortable with that label. If I don't survive, I don't want to feel as if I've somehow failed simply because my word choice didn't come true.

I also don't want to impose a narrative on anyone else by calling them a *warrior* or a *survivor*. So, I've started using the term cancer sojourner—a gentler, more neutral word. A *sojourner* is someone on a journey, moving through a place, not necessarily conquering it, but experiencing it with awareness and, ideally, forward motion.

If you think about it, you'll notice that just using an explicit word like *patient* can subtly reinforce the social role of patient, which is certainly not a slur, but it subtly positions them as kind of one-down in comparison to all the nonpatient "healthy" people. It denies a certain amount of agency to the person.

We can really unintentionally marginalize or "other" people just by referring to them as *patients*. What's really crazy is how we do this to ourselves! If we keep thinking of and referring to ourselves as patients, we focus on our helplessness rather than our strength.

Moreover, if every conversation I have is ninety percent about my cancer experience, I am allowing cancer to be my central identity in the minds of others. When I noticed this, I realized I can shift my identity away from cancer by changing the conversation through the introduction of other topics—other parts of myself, other stories, other joys.

And when every conversation I have is ninety percent about cancer, I'm reinforcing that identity in myself, too, allowing it to eclipse the rest of who I am. I chose to focus more on other identities.

I could do this in conversation with anyone, but I noticed myself doing this unconsciously (and then consciously when I noticed it, lol), with my doctors and nurses. I always told stories and made jokes and talked about linguistics, and I finally realized I was really actively trying to remind those healthcare professionals that I was not just a patient. I am a person. A charming, interesting, adorable person.

They probably found this tedious at times because I talk a lot and that does not promote efficiency, but it does promote a good doctor/patient relationship, which also promotes patient compliance, which promotes treatment success, which promotes doctor satisfaction, so you can see that in the end... everyone wins! I'm not just an egocentric chatterbox—I've got a grand plan for humanity going here.

I also worked on this by reminding myself that I always had something to give, no matter how sick I was. I always asked the nurses about their lives and got into deep conversations with them. Because I also want them to know that I see them as more than their professional identity. I see people who should be noticed and appreciated and amused and encouraged and inspired. So, I made a great effort to connect with every healthcare professional I interacted with.

Moreover, I realized I can make sure I am inhabiting an identity that is much larger than cancer by setting an intention to pursue other activities that are not related to cancer. Certainly, *cancer sojourner is* quite central to one's identity while undergoing treatment. However, I spent many hours every day writing, and that kept my identity as a writer very central in my own mind and I think in the minds of my readers.

I also continued to be a lector at my wonderfully progressive church, performing every Sunday for a Facebook live recorded service for the first nine months or so of the Covid lockdown. In this way, I continued to minister to my beloved congregation and not be reduced to someone who is ministered to by everyone else. That was super important to me. I didn't want to stop loving people in this way.

Furthermore, I chose to continue teaching all the way through chemo and thus was able to retain my professional identity. This is one way that the pandemic actually created an opportunity for me as I could teach all my classes online from my home. At one point, I even taught one class from the hospital!

While I was teaching through Covid, I always dressed professionally on teaching days and wore make-up and jewelry even though I was teaching from home. Taking a shower and putting on makeup and looking nice reminded me that I was still a vibrant, viable human being with many hats (oh, so many hats, after I started losing my hair!)

Just because I have cancer does not mean that I and my cancer have become the center of the universe (I am not sure all my friends agree with this self-assessment, but I did try to keep pouring out to others and not let giving be a one-way street).

I am choosing my identity by my focus and my activity and my language. These are all things I choose. I find that identity construction is a collaborative endeavor. And it can even be a competitive sport as others will keep putting you back in your patient identity and you will have to keep stepping back outside it. Deciding how I want to shape my own identity is one more way that I take cancer's keys (or grief's) away. I tell it, "Get in the back seat, I'm driving."

1. Whorf, Benjamin Lee. *Language, Thought, and Reality: Selected Writings of Benjamin Lee Whorf*. Edited by John B. Carroll, MIT Press, 1956.

2. Tannen, Deborah. *The Argument Culture: Stopping America's War of Words*. Ballantine Books, 1998.

3. Rodgers, Richard, and Oscar Hammerstein II. *I'm Gonna Wash That Man Right Outa My Hair*. *South Pacific*, directed by Joshua Logan, performances by Mary Martin and Ezio Pinza, Majestic Theatre, 1949.

4. Aurelius, Marcus. *Meditations*. Translated by Gregory Hays, Modern Library, 2002.

28

— • —

HOPE MANAGEMENT

Are you a person who wants to know the good, the bad and the ugly about your situation or are you someone who would rather not know if things are not leaning toward a happy ending? It's amazing how differently we each prefer to consume our doses of reality. Some want it straight, some want it diluted, some want a cup of sugar with each teaspoon of truth, and some want to just skip the dose altogether.

Everybody Has Their Own Theory of Hope

Cancer, like many journeys of illness, is a roller coaster. There are a number of factors that contribute to this violent ride. First of all, the goings on in your body are in a constant state of flux. The progress of the disease has unexpected twists and turns. This in itself is enough to make you want to toss your cookies.

Second, every doctor sees something different, which is one reason you want second and third opinions, but is also why the conflicting array of opinions may make you crazy.

Third, I feel like nobody talks about how every doctor has a different philosophy of hope management[1] and, in fact, so does every patient. And since there are so many cooks in the kitchen for a disease like cancer, it makes for potentially questionable hope soup. It is better if you find a recipe you like ahead of time and post it over the stove, so you don't forget your own preferences, metaphorically speaking, in the chaos of conflicting messages.

I learned most of this from my experience with Diane. Some of her doctors wanted her to fight to the death even if she was going to have no quality of life in her final weeks. Others were more compassionate and wanted her to go to palliative care so she could have a better death.

Moreover, some seemed to think that inflating her odds might help her overcome the odds. Others seem to think that not telling her her odds was a better practice so she could exceed expectations.

Just weeks before Diane died, one of her oncologists was still talking as if her stage four stomach cancer could be beat. As one doctor left the room, another entered with a totally different take. Sometimes we saw four different doctors in a day, who all told us something different about what they thought her chances were and what was happening with the disease.

We felt like we were getting whiplash from the differences in opinion—torn between hope, realism, and everything in between.

The antidote to fear is always hope. And hope is not something you pull out of . . . thin air. Hope doesn't just happen to you. You need to happen to hope. You need to find it inside of you and cultivate it. And in order to cultivate it, you have to make choices about various aspects of your situation. One of those is the treatment of information about your health.

When I was in graduate school twenty years before my cancer experience, I had a bunch of weird symptoms, and they were testing me for everything at the Georgetown research hospital, Lupus and MS, among other exciting possibilities.

I had something biopsied on the inside of my thigh, and a female resident asked me, "Do you know why we are so concerned?" I said, "No." She explained in a sympathetic tone, "We are worried that it might be T-Cell Lymphoma." The male resident doing the biopsy blurted out, "Don't tell her that!" *Don't tell me?! What, am I five?!*

His attitude was so insulting to me because I am one of those people who wants to know everything the doctor knows (as, apparently, was the female resident). But on reflection, I realized, not everyone does want to know. And the doctor does not know which sort of person I am. Whether or not he is a good diagnostician, he is surely not clairvoyant. And that is not his fault.

I am convinced that there should be a preliminary survey on what sort of person the patient is, and the results should be in one's file and reviewed by every doctor before every medical encounter. Unfortunately, I do not have institutional reform in the palm of my hand. I do, however, have my words and am perfectly capable of communicating my wishes to said doctor. And now I know that's my responsibility.

The first choice you have in regard to hope management is about how you want your doses of information. Are you a person who wants to know the good, the bad, and the ugly about your situation or are you someone who would rather not know if things are not leaning towards the outcome you had in mind?

It's striking how differently people prefer to receive the truth. Some want it raw and unfiltered, others prefer it softened or sweetened. Some would rather avoid it entirely. And most of us want the autonomy to decide what counts as truth in the first place—which, of course, makes things even trickier.

There are two things you need to be able to do in order to manage your hope regarding the receipt of information. The first is to ask yourself which kind of person you are? Have you thought about how straight you want your information? I urge you to ponder that and find a way to articulate it.

Second, once you figure this out, it's your responsibility to communicate that preference to others (doctors, family, friends, anyone who might be in the grapevine of relevant information). You do not get to be mad because others can't read your mind. You cannot assume that they have the same preferences you have. You must tell them how you want to be communicated with. If you want your needs honored, you have to name them.

Precisely Which Carnival Ride Provides the Best Metaphor

My friend Soncee decided this cancer journey was more of a tilt-a-whirl than a roller coaster, and I am inclined to agree. It shakes you to your bones without the thrill of dead drops (pardon the D word). I had a horrible experience when I was about seven and Eric was about four, and our dad put us on that ride, having no idea it would prove to be an experience of pure terror. They had to stop the ride because we were crying so hard. If only the world worked like that. If only it would stop and let us off when we cry hard enough. If they can't stop the world, it would be nice if doctors could at least be on the same page and stop the dizziness. Unfortunately, you can't herd doctors any more than you can herd cats. That means it comes back to you knowing what your philosophy of hope is. How do you feel about statistics, for instance?

Say they tell you that you have a 30% chance of survival. What percentage are you going to assume you are in? The 70 or the 30? Would you rather not know the statistics or bravely forge ahead with the goal of defying them? Deciding your philosophy of statistics before the deluge can be very liberating.

Knowing your philosophy of hope ahead of time will help you respond to the cacophony of feuding, disputing, or seemingly deluding doctors' opinions. It will help you maintain your equanimity and peace in the midst of the storm.

I am not terrified by cancer, but I am exhausted beyond belief by the shaking and lurching and jerking and feints. The vacillation of urgency levels—do I need to plan my funeral now, or do I have a little while? Do I plan for a crash landing, or can I enjoy a peaceful descent? Cancer wants to drive you off a cliff. Thinking through your philosophy of hope is one way you can kick cancer out of the driver's seat and make sure you're the one behind the wheel.

Let Me Relieve You of a Nagging Uncertainty

And while we are on the topic of hope...

If this has not already happened to you (and I hope it never does, but if you are reading this book, the probability that it has is high, and I am so sorry), you may have this nightmare. You are sitting in the doctor's office, shivering in your skivvies, and those loathsome words come slithering out of her mouth... you have... stage four cancer... (read this word with a hiss).

Even if you are very religious, equally offensive words are very likely to come exploding out of your own mouth. And when the dust settles, you will ask the one question you least want to hear the answer to... *Am I going to die?*

Your whole SHORT (way too short!) life passes before your eyes, and you think, *Wait, what was the point? What is the point of me? Why am I here? Did these few short years matter?*

First of all, I think we can all agree that one of the features of cancer that bites most is the uncertainty. I suppose the younger we are, the more convinced we are that we have some kind of 21st century birthright to certainty. Isn't this the age of science and technology? Doesn't science have cold, hard facts that we can stand on like a rock foundation? I think the older you get, your expectations probably lower with experience.

Nevertheless, when we have a terminal diagnosis, with great confidence and not a little sense of entitlement to knowledge, we tend to ask, "How long do I have?" We are scared to hear the answer, but we also demand it. This is because we crave certainty, which feeds our illusion of control. We apparently believe that medicine is math and should always have a straightforward, unambiguous right answer. Normally, we want our doctors to be really scientifically grounded in cold, hard, both-feet-planted-on-solid-ground facts. We prefer someone who graduated at the top of their class because they have the steely-eyed ability to look at the physical evidence and tell us what the problem is and how to fix said problem.

However, the question itself is a problem because medicine is not math. Anything organic is a little more like the weather—we can predict the weather part of the time to a partial degree of accuracy based on past weather patterns but often get it wrong because Mother Nature apparently gets a kick out of not being predictable.

It's the same way with the human body. That which is organic seems to have a will of its own, a lot like the weather, which does not lend itself towards predictability. As one surgeon told me, almost apologetically, "Medicine is more of an art than a science." Gosh, that's frustrating.

Somehow, this fact, which is kind of obvious on reflection, seems to elude us. And so inevitably we ask, "How long do I have?" as though medicine were either math or mysticism. I think that question has got to be the bane of the existence of every physician who has ever donned a lab coat.

All she can do is compare other cases of a similar cancer with totally different bodies (and minds!) she has seen over the years and guestimate. And to the best of her ability, she offers a tenuous number. And yet the patient tends to receive this number like it was handed down from Mt. Sinai, clinging to it in mad faith.

I know I did. The ER doctor told me I had stage IV pancreatic cancer and I *might* have a year, possibly more with treatment. (He was wrong, but that's a story for another chapter). I immediately began planning my demise based on that timeline.

If the person lives longer than the doctor guessed, this is sometimes treated as a miracle rather than evidence that the doctor miscalculated. If they don't live so long, there is bound to be some anger directed at him. But we give that number so much credence because we so desperately want someone on this earth to be able to tell us the number of our days.

All I want to say is that we need to embrace the uncertainty. Don't cling so tightly to a magic number that isn't actually magic at all. Don't close off the possibility that you might far outlive that number. Be prepared, at the same time, to have to check out a little earlier than you thought.

This is essentially what faith is. Whatever Spirit of life moves in you also requires you to dance with uncertainty. Hope is about knowing you can manage, whatever the outcome. I hope you can find this kind of faith and rest in it, no matter what uncertainty swirls around you.

As for question number one, let me just rip the Band-Aid off for you right here and now. Why, yes. Yes, you are going to die. You are mortal. Maybe today, maybe next year, maybe seventy years from now, you are going to die. Are you going to meet that day prepared to make it as beautiful as possible?

Failure to Plan Ahead

Have you ever made a big sign in permanent marker and gotten to the edge of the page before you finished the last word? Say your wife is coming home from Afghanistan, and you make a Welcome Home sign, but you run out of room for the last two letters, so you have to put the *m* and *e* on the next line, so the first thing she sees is:

Welcome Ho -
me.

Not quite what you were going for. Failure to plan ahead.

The immortal Greek gods were jealous of our mortality because if you're going to live forever, it doesn't really matter what you do today—you can always do it tomorrow or a hundred thousand years from now. But when you are mortal, every moment matters.

Because we none of us know the number of our days, and this fact is exquisitely beautiful like that flower, Queen of the Night, that blooms only once a year in the middle of the night. How much more precious the days that are few. Rarity and scarcity render a thing that much more precious.

False Positivity: The American Thirst for Winning Tells Us Dying Is Losing

As I watched my cherished friend die at the age of thirty, I shook my head helplessly. Who could blame the child for being unprepared? She wanted to live! And she thought she could do so by sheer force of will. She fought like a honey badger, but they discovered her cancer too late. By the time she realized she was dying, she had very little mental clarity left. And she died a very messy, unfinished death. We didn't know what we were doing.

I think Diane was a victim of American positivity culture. Now, don't get me wrong. I am passionate about being positive. But there is naïve positivity and there is realistic positivity. I am a fan of the latter. Naïve positivity can lead you to false conclusions. I would call that *false positivity* (even though doctors would look down their noses at me for the misuse of the term; call it *toxic positivity* if you prefer).

On the other hand, there is plenty of research that shows that anticipating resistance and making a plan to surmount it sets you up for greater success.[2] Hope is vital. But pretending there is no darkness does not lead to light. It only leaves us stumbling when night falls.

Diane grew up in Belgium, but it turns out she was American to the core. Americans want to win above all else (this trait is hilariously highlighted by Melody Moezzi in *The Rumi Prescription*, when she discovers that, in America, competitive yoga is a thing!), and nothing illustrates this thirst to win more than the epic battle of hand-to-hand combat with cancer. It's not just that whoever dies with the least toys loses, as the bumper sticker goes. Whoever *dies* loses!

Death really cramps the American style! I mean, how can you maintain your "I Am the Master of My Own Damned Destiny" myth if you can't even dictate the number of your days? It seems that we have just one gear: In it to win it. And we have decided that dying is not winning.

It is as if many people think that planning for both possible eventualities (living and dying) means you have already given up. If you don't plan your funeral, the thinking seems to be, you won't have to go to it. In my case, I'd rather be prepared and have a hand in planning my funeral and everything surrounding my final transition.

Diane didn't know. She was a victim of the variety of culturally reinforced optimism that refuses to acknowledge we cannot control all outcomes. This can be disastrous.

Hindsight Is 2020

(Heh heh. It was 2020. And I had twenty years of hindsight, so it was 20 20/20 2020. Some kind of very special vision). When I received my own grave diagnosis of stage IV pancreatic cancer, I realized I had to seize the reins.

I felt like I was sitting in the audience watching the humorous speech contestants and rewriting my international Toastmasters speech in my head, when suddenly I was called on stage to perform. *This is it! No more prep time. Whatever you have to give, you have to give it now. Pour out everything you have. This is your last chance.* So, I decided to make my dying a work of art.

I Just Called to Say *I Love You*

If you've never lived in another culture, you probably don't know this but saying "I love you" at the end of every single phone conversation you have with your dear ones is a peculiarly American thing. Most cultures don't do that. When I was living in Japan, I was told you tell your spouse that you love them one time and then that's pretty much good for life. It's like this coupon never expires. I think it's like saying "I do" in your wedding ceremony. It's a speech act, something you do one time and it's good. You don't do it over and over (at least not with the same spouse).

Expressing our affection in words is really important to us here in the States, though. If asked, most Americans explain that just in case the other person dies suddenly, you want the last thing you said to them to have been, "I love you." When people do know they are about to die, they instinctively call their most intimate people so they can tell them one more time, "I love you."

When you know the end is near, you're given a rare gift; you have a little bit of control over your last social, spiritual, and emotional acts.

Are you going to die? Yes. And planning for that eventuality will not hasten its coming. I repeat, making peace with your eventual (and certain) demise will not cause you to die sooner. But it may give you a much more beautiful conclusion. Do you want your life to look like an unfinished sign scribbled by a drunk monkey? Wouldn't you rather plan ahead and make your dying a work of art?

For My Money Realistic Positivity Is the Best Approach to Hope Management

I know that hope management probably sounds like a group of real estate caretakers. Chuckle (that's an imperative. It's ok to chuckle and think about grief at the same time. In fact, highly recommend. You have to come up for air as often as you can. Grief feels like drowning. You need air. Find your air wherever you can). Hope management refers to the fact that hope is something we have to very consciously cultivate by making specific choices. There are so many threats to our hope that we have to respond to intentionally in order to preserve and promote it.

It matters what you do with your last moments. (I apologize to those of you for whom this is obvious, but it wasn't obvious to Diane and there might be others for whom it isn't.) This is your last opportunity to give some gift from your soul to anyone you love.

They will live the rest of their lives never hearing anything else from your heart. What will you give them? What will you leave them with? Having a plan is about a very important kind of hope that lasts beyond the grave. The hope of continuing to give life and encouragement to someone after you are gone. This hope does not disappoint.

---

1. This is my nifty term.

2. Oettingen, Gabriele. Rethinking Positive Thinking: Inside the New Science of Motivation, Current, 2014.

29

— · —

GIFTS OF A DEATH SENTENCE

Mind Blown

On July 9, almost three weeks after my fateful ER visit, about four o'clock in the afternoon, I was sitting under a tall sycamore on the deck having a goodbye conversation with one of my closest friends by Zoom. The weather was gorgeous, my hair was softly blowing in the breeze lovelier than ever (oh hair! Remember hair?), and it was a beautiful, peaceful conversation about bringing my life to a loving close.

The phone rang. It was my general practitioner, so I told my friend I'd call her back. The results of the biopsy had come in. To everyone's astonishment, it was *not* pancreatic cancer! It was *lymphoma* that had metastasized to my pancreas! (There were several good-sized tumors in my pancreas.) I quickly googled lymphoma and found a forty to sixty percent chance of survival! Up from zero! Four doctors had been *dead* certain I had metastatic pancreatic cancer and would be dead in a matter of months.

Learning that you have Stage IV Metastatic Pancreatic Cancer, particularly when you have so long labored under the ludicrous illusion that you were somehow immune to cancer, will blow your head right off your shoulders. Unlearning it after three weeks? Also mind blowing. It seems like there should be a cap on how many times your mind can be blown in just one month. And it's hard to turn on a dime when you thought you were hurtling over a cliff like Thelma and Louise. My head wasn't even spinning. I was just stunned.

I called my mother first and then my closest friends. Some of them burst into tears with relief. I myself was much more tempered in my response. By this time, I was wary of diagnoses and their irksomely volatile changeability. I decided I would take everything with a grain of salt (the size of a truck) for a while. It may be worth noting, I received this news with the same calm I displayed at the original diagnosis.

In a day or two, I saw the oncologist, who told me it was Diffuse Large B-Cell Lymphoma. He thought I had a ninety-five percent chance of survival, but at the time, he didn't realize I had a specific subtype: non-GCB, with bone marrow involvement. Only about fifteen percent of lymphoma patients present with the cancer already in their bones, and that factor, along with my age and other health considerations, brought my actual survival odds down to around seventy percent.

Still, seventy percent felt like a slam dunk by contrast to what I thought I had been facing. If I had a real chance, I would definitely fight for it.

Pshaw

I got into a clinical trial with NIH—the National Institutes of Health—which is only about thirty miles away from where I lived. I had world-class cancer care, and my treatment was all free. I didn't know how I could be more blessed. I know not getting cancer in the first place occurs to some of you, to which I reply with a Dickensian *Pshaw!*

Yes, I am one of those weirdos who claims that cancer is one of the best things that has ever happened to her. Not just cancer. A terminal misdiagnosis is one of the best things that has ever happened to me. I'll admit, I might feel differently if I had died within a year. But even then, I believe the experience would still have made my life more intense, more vivid, and more beautiful. Facing death sharpened my awareness, clarified my values, and opened my heart in ways nothing else ever had.

I can imagine some people might be angry about the emotional suffering caused by a terminal misdiagnosis. I don't feel that way at all. I feel that it was a magnificent gift. Of course, the first and most obvious gift of a terminal misdiagnosis is the elation of having the death sentence lifted.

Stage IV cancer suddenly looks good when you thought you were headed for certain death, and now it's a curable cancer and not one of the deadliest. Chemotherapy looks wonderful when you realize it is very likely going to keep you alive. It was so easy to be cheerful about chemo and cancer with that perspective.

Honestly, I almost think a terminal misdiagnosis followed by a more curable diagnosis could be a strangely powerful prescription for those facing treatment—a radical reframe for those who need help shifting how they see their diagnosis and the prospect of chemotherapy or other treatment options. When you've looked death in the eye and been pulled back, even suffering takes on a different texture.

What I Learned about Myself

To begin with, I learned that I am not afraid of death. I could not have learned that any other way. You can hypothesize about how you would feel until the cows come home, but until it *happens* to you, you simply do not know. I thought I would be afraid. I was stunned to discover I was not. There is a great peace that comes with this realization. I also learned that I am much stronger than I knew. That is good to know. I assume that it will serve me well in the many years to come.

Remember that day when I started throwing all my books in boxes and clearing out my room to make it all invalid friendly? Reading books can be a very future oriented activity. You can read because you are filling your brain with knowledge to be used at another time. As an academic, that has been a prevailing view for me.

Getting a terminal diagnosis where the future became irrelevant, I felt like Lewis and Clark discovering an exotic place called *Here and Now*. Knowledge is intrinsically pleasurable, so I'm going to keep reading. Living in the moment sets you free from being completely utilitarian.

After my experience helping Diane die and before my own diagnosis, I regularly maintained that there are no bad days. Every day I wake up is a *good* day. After cancer, I felt even more poignantly that every day is a special occasion. Have the steak. Use the crystal. Eat the raspberries. Walk barefoot in the grass. Say yes to what gives you joy. Eat, drink, and be merry. You will pass this way but once.

Every day is dappled with moments of pain and moments of joy. In a paraphrase of Rumi's words, *Grief and unexpected joy live in a doorway where there is no time or distance.*[1] They are both standing there. You can find beauty and meaning in entertaining them both. In fact, so many moments are undecided, only good or bad as thinking makes them so. Sift out all those beautiful moments and savor them.

For me, this new focus on dwelling in the moment didn't mean I intended to throw the future completely out the window just because I was dying. I was still thinking about the future of my loved ones and how I could weasel my way into it by way of burying myself deep in their hearts and memories long after I am physically no longer with them. I wanted to be a joyful, beautiful memory. I wanted somehow for my life to continue to feed their souls, even after I was gone.

There was such urgency. I was so afraid that I wasn't going to have time to leave each loved one with an understanding of just how important they were to me. It was very interesting that once that time limit was lifted and I was given a reprieve, I stopped working on some of those things.

After some weeks, I realized, now that I have (presumably) all this time, let me get to it. Let me not procrastinate in showing my loved ones how much I love them. Write the poems and the letters. Have the conversations. Make the revelations. Chop, chop!

What Have I Done with My Life?

Another thing that I also realized is that I am happy with what I have done with my life, even though by the standards of many, I am far from a success. I never put much stock in money or material possessions. I put my stock in nourishing souls. I am happy with the investments I have made in that regard.

By the time of my complete resurrection in 2019, I realized two things. First, there is one great blessing in being fifty-plus years old and not having a partner, and that is that this is the only way you can know for sure that you are 100 percent complete in yourself. I have not been super impressed by the average marriage. I have embraced the wisdom that it is better to be single and lonely than married and lonely. (Although I am not lonely at all). I am also pleased that whenever someone asks my mother if Elisa is married yet, she always says, "No and she's not divorced yet either."

Second, one day I posted on Facebook: *I am congratulating myself for all the men who are still alive because I did not marry them.* I really think that might be the funniest (and truest?) thing I have ever said. I have seen a lot in the husbands of my friends that make me think, if a man said that to me, one day he just would not wake up. (Oh, come on, that's hysterical. Don't look so horrified).

When I was fifty-three, I was still dreaming of finding a soulmate, but I did not feel incomplete. I did not need such a person to make me happy. I found that I was complete in my own damned self, and I'm not sure that I could have known that if I had not been single all my life. And learning that I was going to die without ever having found that person was not particularly tragic. Because my life was full of love. I have so many rich, intimate relationships. I have more intimate relationships with my friends than I see many having with their spouses. I am content.

I am perfectly happy without money, without a romantic partner, without wild professional success, without so many things that so many believe their happily ever after must be predicated upon.

Different View of Possessions

My friend Dee bought me a beautiful red leather tote (which I picked out) early in my cancer journey which I was going to hashtag #ChemoChic, but which my more spiritually minded friend hashtagged #SacredObject. This idea of objects being made sacred by gifting them helped change my view of my possessions.

As I walked through my apartment and made plans for who would get each prized possession—I mean, who was going to get all my new size 8 dresses?? (Understand that when you were a 16 the year before, that makes them super precious). That weighed heavily on my mind <insert mirthful ironic smile>. I found that I had a different view of those things that I owned. I started thinking in terms of sacred objects.

When I began to contemplate to whom I would give each item and what it would mean to them, I realized that a lot of things that I have would bring me more happiness if I gave them away to people who are precious to me. After my diagnosis changed and it appeared that I would live, I continued to think of how much more happiness certain items would give me if I presented them to a loved one. I gave gold rings to two dear friends because I wanted them to know *before* I died how much they mean to me.

Fifteen Minutes of Fame

Not everyone enjoys the limelight, but I do. When you have a terminal diagnosis, your life is the proverbial train wreck that people can't look away from. When it looked like I was going to expire imminently, I found that people cared more than usual about what I had to say. They were listening. So, I tried to share everything important that I had in my soul. That led to my blog, which ultimately led to this book, another gift of cancer. Having the occasion and the purpose to write it was a gift. The pleasure of writing it was a gift to me, and I hope the result will be a gift to my readers.

Love Pouring Out of the Universe: Relationships Restored to Me

Perhaps the most precious gift of a terminal diagnosis was to learn that I am even more deeply loved by even more people than I knew. There is a beautiful proverb in the Old Testament, "A friend loveth at all times and a brother is born for adversity."[2] Times of crisis and trauma are such wonderful opportunities for us to show our love to one another.

I was so touched by the outpouring of love I received from people right here and from all over the world, which made me realize without a doubt that I am extremely wealthy in my friends. People cooked and baked and gave me money and gifts and flowers and edible arrangements. They drove me to my appointments, some of them self-isolated for me, Mike and Tina even bought me groceries for six months and delivered them straight to my refrigerator, all Cloroxed down to make sure covid didn't touch me.

One of the greatest gifts of my terminal diagnosis was the restoration of several important friendships with people I have deeply loved but had grown apart from over the years, just because life took us to other parts of the globe. A few of these friends I hadn't seen in thirty or forty years, but when they found out about my stage IV cancer, they were right there, loving me and walking with me through this scary time. They all threatened to get on a plane immediately upon learning of my diagnosis, but it was the beginning of the covid pandemic, and we didn't have a vaccine yet, so I politely told them to stay the heck away, at least until we had a vaccine or I was just a couple of weeks from death.

My dear friend Hiroko began making plans to come from Japan to care for me in my final weeks. It was a priceless gift to me to know that she would do this for me. And now these friends continue to be right here with me, even though the danger is past. For the restoration of any one of these relationships, the whole cancer journey would have been worthwhile.

I also made some brand-new friends through cancer. I was further blessed by so many nurses I never would have met without cancer. They enriched my life, and I hope that I enriched theirs. I also found there were a couple of people who really didn't care that I was dying, and that was super clarifying. It was painful, but I was able to let go of them.

I believe that when you put love out into the universe, it will come back to you, though it won't always come back to you from the same people.

I Gained a Mother, My Own

Quite remarkably, through cancer, my mother and my sister found their compassion for me, and it completely changed the way my mother talks to me. It made me wonder how our relationship might be different if she had always spoken to me with such tenderness. I just think that if she had always talked to me the way she talks to me now, we would have had a much more beautiful relationship. I'm so blessed to have her restored to me. This cancer would have all been worthwhile just to have my mother back after 50 years. I am so grateful.

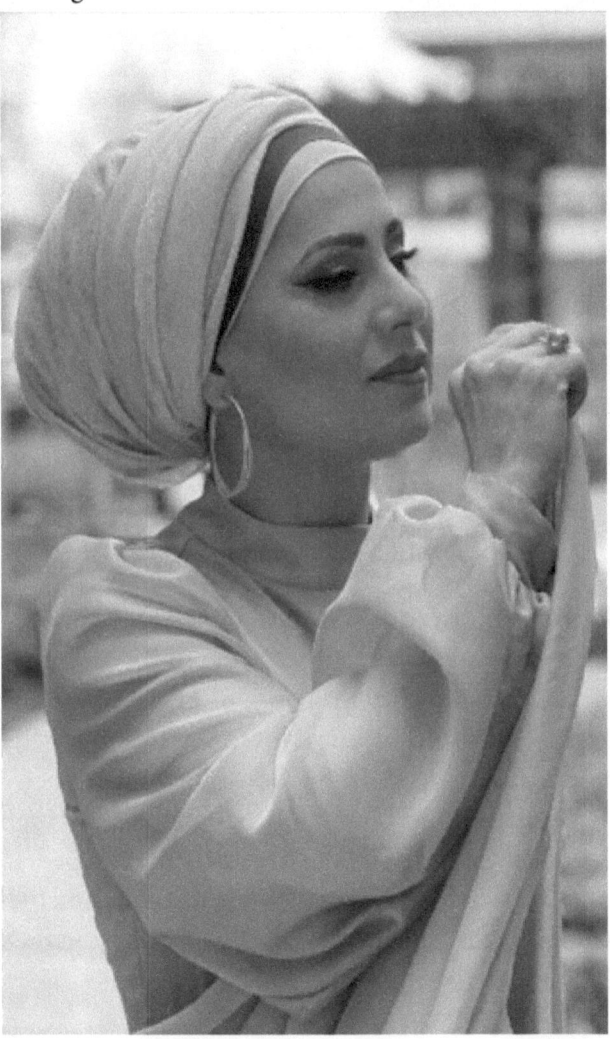

My Daughter, Malalai

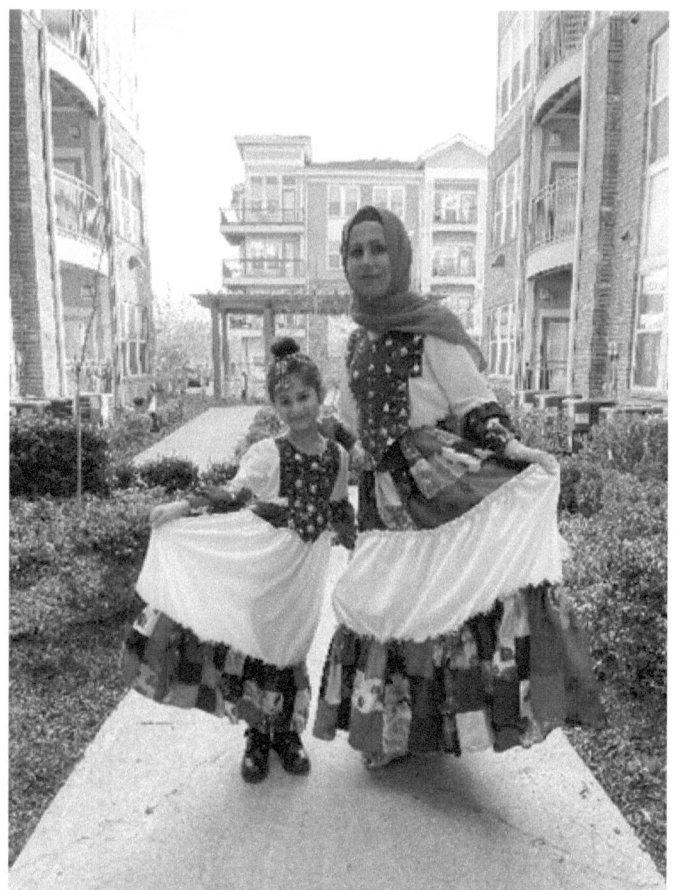

My Granddaughter, Asnah, and Malalai

I Gained a Daughter (and a Granddaughter)

Diane's cancer was an opportunity for me to lay down my life for her for a few months and show her the depth of my love (You remember she exclaimed to me, "I had no idea you loved me this much.") The cancer provided an opportunity to show her how much I loved her. In the same way, my dear Malalai, whom I have since adopted as my daughter, offered to quit her job and drop out of school to care for me as I died. If I had never had this diagnosis, I would never have known just how much she loved me. Again, the whole cancer journey would have all been worthwhile for even that one priceless revelation.

Don't Think This is Over, Grim!

June 27, 2020

Okay, this might make me sound sick, twisted, or possibly just an especially committed emo goth—but part of me kind of regrets that I didn't get the chance to see it all the way through. To test the theory. To prove that it's possible to grieve joyfully right to the end. Not because I'm in denial, but because I *really* wanted to know if this could be done. I wanted to be living proof.

For years, I've longed to help people, especially my dearest ones, grieve better. Facing death would've been the ultimate opportunity to model that. But... sigh. I guess I'll just write a book. Everything in its time. Make no mistake: I don't want a short life. But I *do* love a challenge. It's like training for the Olympics only to have the games canceled because of some dumb pandemic.

So, since there is a high possibility of beating this cancer, TRUST, I WILL KICK ITS ASS. No ifs, ands, or butts (heh heh) about it. I do solemnly promise. (But not too solemn... there must always be laughter, especially in the darkness).

And to Death I say,
Don't think this is over, Grim!
I know you will come for me one day
and I will be ready for you then, too!

The Effect of Curable Cancer vs. Terminal Cancer on Your Relationships

A curious thing happened when my death sentence was lifted. Some of the dear ones who had returned, who had shown up with their whole hearts after years of distance, faded away again once it became likely I would live. I don't blame them. But I did feel the loss.

I don't know what it is about the intimacy of imminent death, but it's real. With a terminal diagnosis, time with you is at a premium that it will lose when your life expectancy expands. And it is in that scarcity that beauty shines most brightly.

There is oh so much beauty there in the shadow of imminent death and I believe that it is in that holy light that the scales fall from your eyes, and you can see clearly that love truly is the only thing that matters. I think that's what draws people in. When death becomes less imminent, the pull subsides.

In fact, as I have said, each one of those relationships is a treasure and I consider my whole cancer journey an absolutely fair exchange. As it is, I feel I won the lottery.

So, as for those three weeks of misdiagnosis, I regret nothing. On the contrary, I am absolutely filled with gratitude. I was given a magnificent gift that will shine a bright and holy light on the rest of my life. My heart will sing a song of thanksgiving all my days (however few or many they turn out to be).

If I could create an animated gif to go right here, it would look like this: The Grim Reaper is standing there in his holocaust cloak looking down. But as he lifts his head, you see the face of the angel of death is radiant. He spreads his arms and his cloak opens, and you see piles of beautiful gifts. The shadow of death is not black or even monochrome. It's technicolor.

Therefore, as for that death sentence, I have no regrets about getting stage four cancer or my misdiagnosis. In fact, highly recommend. If I had it to do over, if I could go back in time and decide to skip it, I would absolutely order again. I have gained so much more than I have lost.

Cancer Cornucopia

For any one of these gifts, the cancer would have been worthwhile. To have the gifts pile up like they did I feel that cancer has blessed me with unspeakable riches.

I know that's not true for everyone. For some, cancer is only suffering—no silver linings, no redemptive arc. I don't pretend that my experience speaks for theirs. But this is what was true for me. And I count it among the great miracles of my life.

---

1. Rumi. *Selected Poems by Rumi*. Translated by Coleman Barks with John Moyne, A.J. Arberry, and Reynold Nicholson, Penguin Books, 2004.

2. Proverbs 17:17.

MORE THAN A HAPPY ENDING

"*Let me fall if I must fall. The one I am becoming will catch me.*"
—Attributed to Baal Shem Tov[1]

Ringing the Bell

In some hospitals there is a tradition of ringing a bell when someone has their last chemotherapy treatment. It's a moment of joy, of triumph—a ritual that signals: *You made it. You're done. You're on your way.*

There is no bell for emotional healing. There is no clear point where treatment is finished, and you are "on your way."

I could have rung a bell for the day I sang my song on Brian's grave, but I didn't walk away from that experience a new woman. It was a moment of healing, but there was still convalescence and recuperation to do and that took me a lot longer than may have been necessary. I kind of wish I had a bell to ring now, though. I have reached a stage that's worth ringing for. I'll consider this book to be my bell.

From Blob to Blossom

The real resurrection work of evolving from blob to blossom took place between 2015 and 2019. If I had known then what I know now, I feel sure I could have resurrected much sooner. In Chapter Two, I asked you how you managed your journey from birth to this moment. You now have a pretty good idea how I did, and it wasn't pretty (well, there was beauty along the way, but it was a lot more grueling than it probably needed to be).

Remember that collaborative culinary throwdown we talked about in the beginning? I acknowledged that there are a bunch of ingredients in our lives that we don't get to choose. But the good news is that there is a huge number of ingredients you can absolutely choose, and to your taste. I also promised you snacks. These snacks are not like a juice box and a bag of chips, however. They are going to take some fairly intense preparation. But how divine will be the final product.

Just to recap, here are the ingredients I used to make a tasty meal out of my life even though I was given some very questionable fare to work with. Is it instant? Nope. Is it full of exotic ingredients you've never heard of? Nope. Is it full of superfoods that will transform your life? Absofreakinglutely.

My first critical ingredient was finding a trauma therapist. To this, I added community, spiritual practice, rewriting my inner narrative, transforming my mind with positivity, reading like my soul depended on it, practicing gratitude, setting goals, serving others, and reveling in creativity. If you've ever eaten that fabulous Thai soup Tom Kha Gai, this soup is as delicious as that.

So, if you're still in the blob stage—God bless it. Lie there. Rest. Breathe. But when the moment comes, when you feel the faintest call to rise, even if you think you can't... know that resurrection is not a one-time event. It's a long, slow becoming. It's a choice you make every day. You're allowed to begin small. Maybe one breath. Maybe one book. Maybe one act of kindness to yourself.

Start Telling the Story

Of course, ingredients don't do much good if they just sit on the counter. At some point you have to pick one up and start cooking. Healing is like that too—there comes a time to begin putting your story into motion.

If you've lost someone and don't remember grieving, you probably didn't. It's a memorable experience.

I recommend you find a good therapist. I recommend you talk to someone about the person you lost and the event that took their life.

I also recommend you write. Write letters to your lost loved ones. Write journal pages. This book includes discussion questions at the end that may serve as prompts. Write to someone else you love about the person you lost. Write a poem. A song. Paint something. Move something. Create something.

Just do something to express and externalize your grief—so you can start getting it out of your bones.

Do something to tell your story. Telling—and more importantly, retelling—your story is the beginning of healing.

Bring your wounds into the light of day, where healing may begin.

I'll be over here, cheering you on.

May you discover your own resurrection. Whatever fare life has handed you, I believe you can make something nourishing and luminous from it. I believe your story matters. Your healing matters. And the world is aching for the gifts that only you can bring. If something in these pages lit even the smallest candle in your darkness, then my work here is done. Take what resonates. Leave the rest. Add your own ingredients. Adjust to taste. But please—don't forget to feed your soul. Don't forget the snacks.

---

1. This quote is widely attributed to the Baal Shem Tov, the 18th-century founder of Hasidic Judaism, though no primary Jewish textual sources support that attribution. It more likely originates with Sheryl Sandberg, COO of Facebook and author of *Option B*, who used similar language in public reflections on grief and resilience.

Epilogue

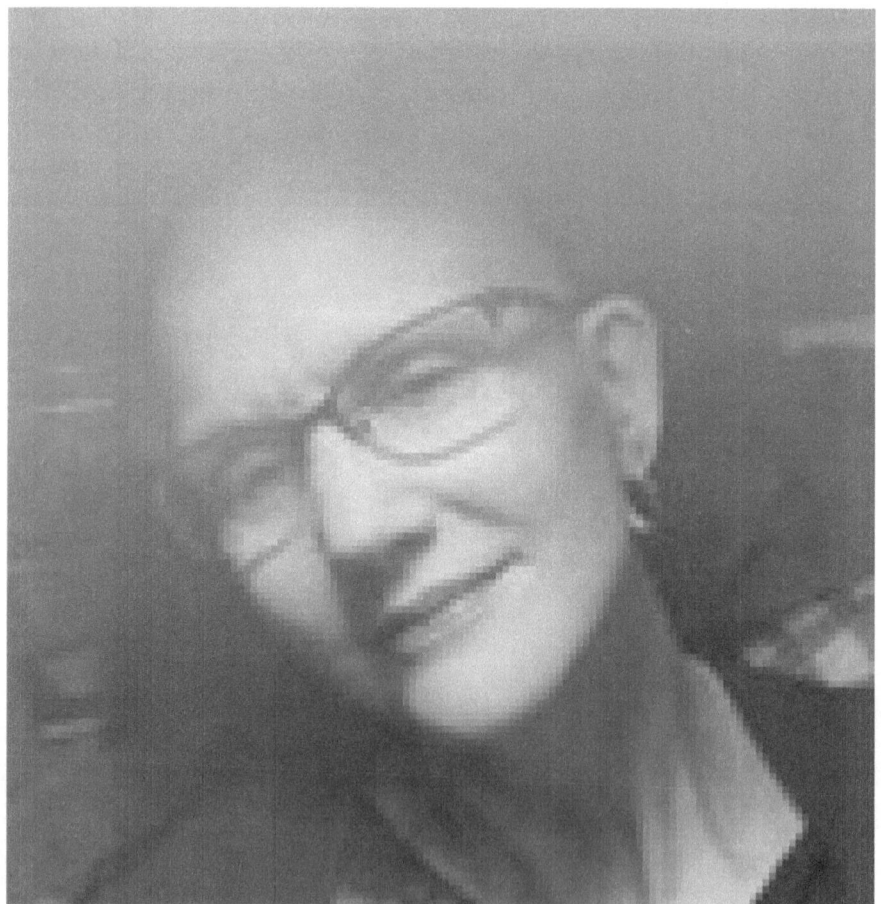

Bald Me. This picture conveniently camouflages my cone headed scalp.

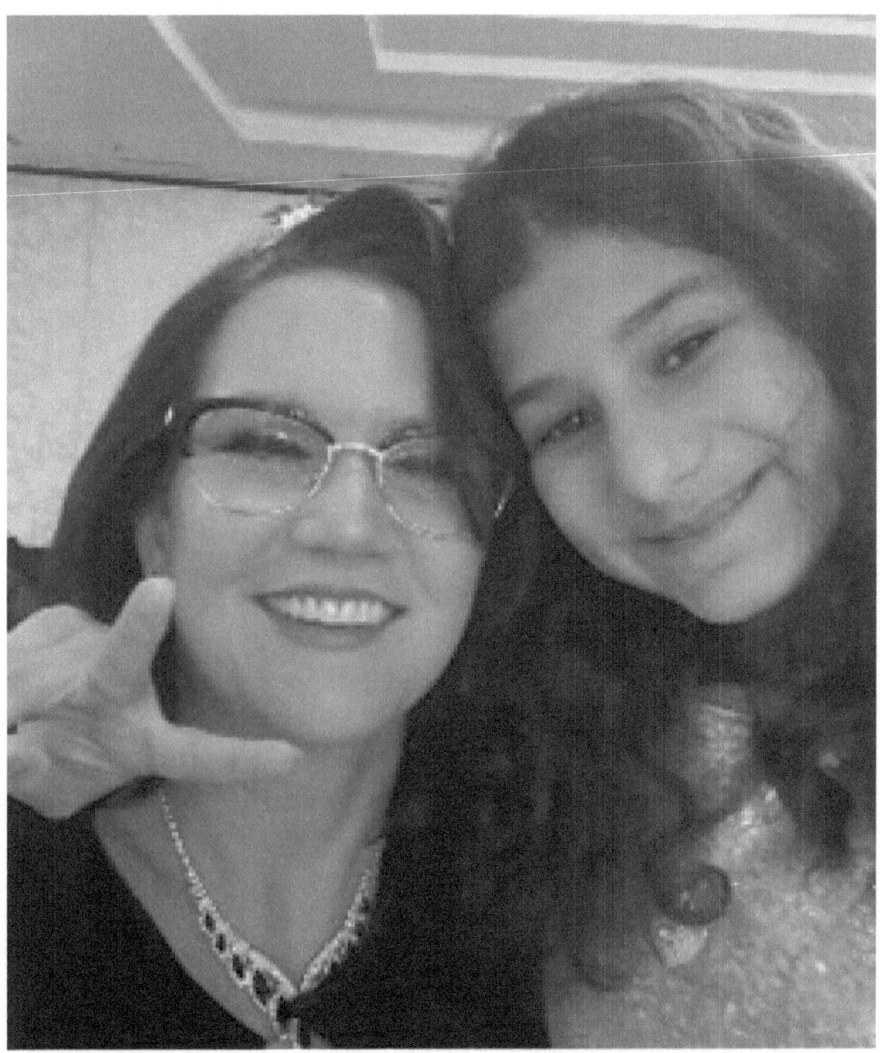

Me and Asnah (2024)

After an experimental drug failed, I went on to undergo EPOCH-R chemotherapy at the National Institutes of Health (since I had a 70% chance of surviving, I was quite happy to accept treatment). My friends took amazing care of me during that time (making the best of living through covid without a vaccine yet).

Chemo was very challenging, and I was hospitalized for a week with 33/60 blood pressure and horrendous and unexplainable vertigo that made me walk like a wildly drunken sailor, but I thanked God every day for chemotherapy. On November 19, 2020, I was declared officially cancer free. In May of 2025 I was told by NIH it would be ok to use the word "cured"! Now I try to strike a balance between planning for a very long life and staying prepared for it to come to completion at any time. But the upshot is this:

I am still here. Not because I deserve to be. Not because I fought harder than anyone else. I'll leave the whys to those wiser than me.

But I'm still here—still raving about the joy of bare feet in the grass, still savoring the raspberries, still marveling at my daughter's smile and letting my granddaughter make me laugh until I cry.

Cancer didn't wake me up. I was already awake.

By the time I got cancer in 2020, I had already healed. In so many ways I had died with Brian and Diane. But I found my resurrection. Somehow healing from their deaths prepared me to meet my own—with peace and even joy. I approached my death not with fear, but with the joy of someone who has truly lived—even if for too short a time.

For life is not beautiful because it is long, Beloveds. It is beautiful because it is deep, full of love, full of joy and full of grace. Death, I've come to believe, can be the final beautiful chapter in a beautiful life.

Of course there is grief. Wherever there is love and beauty, there will be grief. But when I received my terminal diagnosis, I was already whole. I was already full of joy. And I believe it was that joy that helped me carry the grief with a grace that surprised even me. For me, cancer wasn't a crucible, it was confirmation. It was my proof of life.

I don't believe God sent me cancer to test me. But it was a test just the same. And I'm so ridiculously grateful to say: I tested positive—for life.

My cancer proved to me that my long resurrection was complete.

We all have a terminal diagnosis. Even if you're the first to make it to 140 years, your story will end. You may, like me, have been broken beyond recognition. You may, like me, have had times when you begged God to take your life. What I want to leave you with is this: Healing happens. But it doesn't happen just because time passes. It takes work. It takes intention. I won't lie to you; it's a painful process. It may require feeling all the pain again (like having a bone rebroken). But this pain is a healthy, holy, healing pain. Rebirth, like birth, is painful. But—oh my God— the glory of resurrection! I wish you healing. I wish you resurrection. I wish—more than anything—that you would wake before you die.

— • —

DISCUSSION GUIDE

*I**Should Wake Before I Die** by Elisa L. Everts*

This discussion guide was created to encourage reflection, relationship-enriching group conversations, and deeper personal exploration for readers of *I Should Wake Before I Die: Field Notes from the Valley of the Shadow (with Snacks!)*.

Whether you're reading this during illness, in grief, alongside a friend, or simply to remember what it means to truly live, these prompts are here to nourish dialogue and meaning-making. Grab your journal or dedicate a new one to these reflections. It's so easy to read a book and not be changed. Why not do the reflection that will bring more lasting transformation (either alone or in a group, with souls you trust)?

Preface – Before the Valley
Summary:
In this intimate preface, Elisa welcomes readers into sacred space, grief's valley, offering companionship, irreverent humor, and radical honesty. She acknowledges that her story is uniquely hers, shaped by devastating losses and surprising light. Without claiming universal truths or tidy endings, she offers witness and solidarity. This book was born from questions, not answers, from the ache of love that persists beyond death. Above all, she hopes readers feel less alone as they walk through their own shadows.

Discussion Questions:
1. What brought you to this book? Is there a particular loss, struggle, or longing you're carrying right now?

2. Who are the people whose deaths you will never be "at peace" with? How does their love continue to live in you?

3. Do you use humor as a coping tool? How has laughter, especially in dark moments, helped you survive?

4. How do you feel about the idea that light can still show up in the valley of the shadow of death? Have you ever experienced a moment like that?

5. What do you need from a grief companion, whether a person or a book? Can you name what kind of witness you long for?

6. How do you feel when someone talks about God or spirituality in the context of grief? What feels comforting, and what doesn't?

Introduction – Just in Case You Don't Buy This Book

Summary:

In this heartfelt and unflinchingly honest introduction, Elisa offers readers a seed of wisdom upfront: *Life is not beautiful because it is long, but because it is deep and full of love.* She situates the book not as a traditional cancer memoir, but as a soulful journey through grief, healing, and the reclamation of joy. With humor, candor, and warmth, she dismantles tired cultural narratives about illness and survival, offering instead a story of spiritual authorship and radiant agency. Readers are invited not only to witness Elisa's story, but to locate their own light within it, especially in seasons when it feels extinguished.

Discussion Questions:

1. Elisa writes, "Life is not beautiful because it is long...but because it is deep." What does a "deep life" mean to you? Can you name a moment in your life that felt deep rather than long?

2. How has grief (yours or someone else's) shaped the way you view your purpose in life? Do you resonate with the idea that grief can be both devastating and transformative?

3. What role does humor play in your own coping strategies? Did the "Hold my beer" reference shift your perspective on how someone can face mortality?

4. The chapter challenges the idea that someone "loses" a battle with cancer if they die. How do you feel about that narrative? What alternative metaphors or frameworks for illness resonate more deeply with you?

5. Elisa writes about pitching a tent in the Valley of the Shadow of Death and mapping the underworld. What metaphors would you use to describe your own journey through grief, illness, or fear?

Chapter 1 – One Key to Them All

Summary:

In this chapter, Elisa reflects on how profound grief, especially unresolved childhood loss, shaped her ability to face a terminal cancer diagnosis with peace. She argues that emotional resurrection must precede physical death, and that ungrieved sorrow can block spiritual and emotional healing. With raw honesty, she traces her journey through losses, including the death of her baby brother and best friend, and how healing those wounds allowed her to greet mortality with clarity and grace. This is a story about waking up before dying, emotionally, spiritually, and relationally, and reclaiming agency through storytelling, therapy, and fierce, redemptive love.

Discussion Questions:

1. Have you ever experienced a grief so early in life that you didn't realize it was grief until years later?

2. In what ways has childhood loss or trauma shaped how you respond to grief as an adult?

3. Do you carry any grief that feels tangled up with guilt? If so, how has that affected your healing process?

4. What part of your identity felt like it "died" after a loss, and how have you worked (or not yet worked) to reclaim or reshape it?

5. Elisa writes about spending nearly 20 years in the "Valley of the Shadow." How long did your grief feel like it owned your story?

6. What forms of expression—writing, art, conversation—have helped you begin to process and externalize your grief?

Chapter 2 – Who Is Writing Our Stories?

Summary:

This chapter invites readers to reflect on the unpredictable, often painful, often wondrous path of life. With humor, honesty, and spiritual depth, Elisa recounts her own journey—from trauma, loss, and cancer to the liberating realization that she is not merely a character in her story but its co-author. Drawing on metaphor, theology, and poetry, she explores agency, suffering, and the power of reframing our narratives. Life may hand us ingredients we never asked for, but we can still create a nourishing, meaningful feast. This chapter is a tender invitation to reclaim authorship, meaning, and joy—even amid grief.

Discussion Questions:

1. When in your life have you felt like a character in someone else's story? What shifted when you began to reclaim authorship of your own narrative?

2. What are some of the "non-negotiable" plot points in your life story? How have you made meaning from them—or how might you begin to?

3. Have you ever tried to live a "fairy tale" life or skipped to the happy ending in your imagination? What did that attempt reveal about your desires or your wounds?

4. Which voices—cultural, familial, religious—have tried to narrate your life for you? Which ones are you ready to challenge, edit, or silence?

5. Have you experienced a moment when your own story unexpectedly nourished or illuminated someone else's path? What did that reveal about the value of your journey?

6. If you were to name the "crop" you're growing in the secret garden of your heart right now, what would it be—and how can you help

it thrive?

Chapter 3 – Smacked Upside the Head with a Cancer Stick

Summary:

In *Blind Date with the Grim Reaper*, Elisa recounts the seismic shock of a terminal cancer diagnosis in the prime of her life—a moment she describes as a "deathquake." From a place of deep joy and purpose, she is suddenly thrust into crisis, recalling past traumas, especially the sacred and harrowing death of a beloved friend. Yet, rather than surrender to despair, she draws on years of grief, healing, and inner resilience. This chapter introduces her radical decision to live her final chapter as art—loving boldly, writing truthfully, and walking through the dark with light already stored in her soul.

Discussion Questions:

1. Have you ever experienced a "lifequake"—an event that changed everything in an instant? How did it reshape your path or perspective?

2. What do you believe about preparing for death—emotionally, spiritually, relationally? How prepared do you feel right now?

3. Elisa describes having "pre-grieved" through earlier losses. Can grief you've already lived through make future losses more bearable? Why or why not?

4. How do you respond to her idea of making a "final chapter" into a work of art or love? What might that look like for you?

5. Have you ever tried to find meaning or beauty in a moment of crisis or suffering? What helped—or didn't help—at the time?

6. Elisa began a blog as both communication and connection. Have you ever turned to writing, art, or social media during grief or illness? What was the result?

Chapter 4 – Your Number Is Up

Summary:

In this reflective and poetic chapter, Elisa contemplates mortality after receiving a shocking stage IV cancer diagnosis at age 53—decades sooner than expected. She recalls childhood assumptions about longevity and shares a blog post, "Loving Life to the Very Last Drop," which reframes dying as an invitation to live fully. The chapter interweaves present-tense insights with past experiences, including a near-drowning at age five, to illustrate her lifelong awareness of life's fragility. Through humor, poetry, and memory, she embraces her shortened timeline as a sacred opportunity to savor beauty, create meaning, and live each day as art.

Discussion Questions:

1. What age have you always imagined living to? Where do you think that expectation came from?

2. How has your understanding of mortality shifted as you've aged?

3. What metaphors for aging or dying, like "over the hill" or "downhill slope," have shaped your view of life's trajectory?

4. Have you ever experienced a brush with death that made you reevaluate your life? What changed afterward?

5. What helps you stay awake to the "number of your days"? What distracts you from it?

6. Do you resonate more with the idea of "The End" or "The Completion"? Why?

Chapter 5 – Hide and Watch

Summary:

In this chapter, Elisa reflects on the deep well of resilience that allowed her to face a terminal cancer diagnosis with surprising calm. Tracing her emotional strength back through a childhood shaped by trauma, poverty, and loss, she reveals how adversity became both her crucible and her training ground. With fierce humor and candid vulnerability, she explores the cost of grief, the gift of hopeful Pentecostalism, and the fierce grit modeled by her blind mother and imaginative father. What emerges is a portrait of hard-earned emotional fortitude—and a powerful reminder that healing, humor, and hope can coexist with heartbreak.

Discussion Questions:

1. Do you relate to the concept of building strength "brick by brick from the rubble"? What are some of the bricks you've used to build your own inner fortitude?

2. Elisa writes that dying is not the worst thing—feeling responsible for someone else's death is. What are the griefs in your life that feel heaviest, and why?

3. The chapter explores the idea that adversity can prepare us for future challenges. In what ways has your own suffering shaped your ability to meet hardship today?

4. Where did you learn hope? Who taught you that healing or transformation was possible?

5. What beliefs about your own limitations have you outgrown—or want to outgrow?

Chapter 6 – How Could Anyone Grieve for 50 Years?

Summary:

In this harrowing yet ultimately hopeful chapter, Elisa breaks open the anatomy of deep, long-lasting grief by exploring four overlapping types: disenfranchised, complicated, traumatic, and early childhood grief. Through personal testimony, she demonstrates how each of these forms of grief took root in her body and soul—starting with her brother Brian's death in childhood and intensifying after the loss of her close friend Diane. She describes how these invisible wounds became embedded in her nervous system, altered her development, and left her fighting to survive through anxiety, chronic pain, depression, and emotional disorientation. But this chapter is not just about despair—it's a map toward hope. With time, therapy, and spiritual grit, she found healing. This chapter reminds us that no grief is too long or too deep to be healed.

Discussion Questions:

1. Which of the four grief types discussed—disenfranchised, complicated, traumatic, or early childhood—feels most resonant to your own story? Why?

2. Have you ever experienced a kind of pain that felt "invisible" to others? How did that affect your ability to grieve or heal?

3. How has grief affected your body, your nervous system, or your physical health?

4. Have you ever struggled to advocate for yourself in grief? What made it difficult—or what might empower you now?

5. How has your faith, spirituality, or meaning-making been shaped (or shaken) by grief?

6. What hope do you carry (or long to carry) for healing, even if your grief has lasted years or decades?

Chapter 7 – Dying Together

Summary:

This chapter traces Elisa's deep friendship with Diane, whose gruesome death from stomach cancer became the emotional template for Elisa's own experience with terminal diagnosis. Through retrospective letters and raw reflection, Elisa explores themes of soulful companionship, spiritual transformation, and the heartbreak of growing apart before uniting again in grief. Diane's death shattered Elisa yet also served as a kind of "dying before dying," a preparation for facing mortality with courage. The chapter tenderly asks whether it's possible to die with someone without physically dying and affirms the healing power of walking with someone to the edge.

Discussion Questions:

1. Have you ever walked alongside someone you loved as they were dying? What did that experience teach you about life—or yourself?

2. How do your past encounters with death or serious illness shape

your current views on mortality and medical treatment?

3. Can you relate to the idea of "dying before you die"? What attachments, beliefs, or identities have you had to release in your own journey?

4. Do you find it more comforting to face hard truths, or to hold on to hope—even if it's unrealistic?

5. In moments of crisis, do you tend to confront, avoid, or try to fix what's happening? Why?

6. How do your spiritual beliefs—whether religious or not—inform how you think about death, dying, and companionship in death?

Chapter 8 – Cherry Blossoms

Summary:

This chapter explores how mortality sharpens our perception, urging us to notice what matters most. Through intimate letters to her dying friend Diane, Elisa reflects on how cherry blossoms—fleeting and beautiful—mirror the preciousness of life and connection. The chapter weaves moments of academic achievement, spiritual epiphany, and grief, culminating in a call to cherish loved ones *now*. It challenges readers to express deep love before it's too late, to recognize heaven in human form, and to resist letting sacred relationships slip away. It's a meditation on presence, beauty, impermanence, and the holy urgency of telling our beloveds just how much we love them.

Discussion Questions:

1. Have you ever experienced a moment—like Elisa under the cherry blossom tree—that made you suddenly aware of life's fleeting beauty?

2. What losses or transitions have helped you see the importance of living in the present?

3. Is there someone in your life who might not fully know how deeply you love them? What holds you back from telling them?

4. What do you make of the metaphor comparing people to "heaven" placed in our path?

5. How do you typically respond to loss—by clinging more tightly, pulling away, or something else?

6. If you knew you had one year left to live, what would you do differently in your relationships starting today?

Chapter 9 – Falling into a Great Wound

Summary:

This chapter recounts the harrowing final months of Diane's life through the eyes of her friend and caregiver. With raw honesty, the narrator describes the emotional toll of loving someone through terminal illness, the trauma of inadequate support, and the sacredness of presence at the edge of death. It exposes how our culture often abandons the dying and glorifies distance over discomfort. This chapter is both a lament and a testimony—of love that shows up, of friendships tested and remade, and of the great, gaping wound that grief can leave in a soul when someone beloved slips away too soon.

Discussion Questions:

1. How do you personally respond to suffering—your own or others'? Do you retreat, show up, freeze, take charge?

2. Can you recall a time when you were deeply disappointed by others' lack of support in a moment of crisis? How did you process or heal from that?

3. What does it mean to you to "bump the bed" in a relationship—to hurt someone unintentionally while trying to love them? How do you make peace with that?

4. Elisa writes that she felt called to sit with people in the dark. Have you ever felt a similar calling? What does "sitting in the dark" look like in your life?

5. How do cultural or religious expectations shape our ability—or

inability—to ask for help when we're suffering?

6. What does this chapter reveal about who we often see as "family" and the roles non-biological relationships play at the end of life?

Chapter 10 – Not Until Check Out Time

Summary:

In this intimate, reflective chapter, Elisa explores the profound meaning of a life cut short, revisiting the death of her beloved friend Diane to illuminate questions that haunt the living: What makes a life worthwhile? Does length equal value? Through caregiving, spiritual dialogue, and fierce love, Elisa finds clarity in the crucible of loss. These lessons prepared her, years later, to face her own terminal diagnosis with peace. She argues that life is not beautiful because it is long, but because it is full of love, depth, and presence—and that true hope holds, even in the face of death.

Discussion Questions:

1. Have you ever wrestled with the question of what gives your life meaning? How has that understanding changed over time?

2. Do you believe a life must be long to be full? What examples in your life challenge or confirm that belief?

3. How do you respond when someone you love is in denial about their illness or suffering?

4. What does "true hope" mean to you? Does it depend on outcomes, or something deeper?

5. Elisa says, "You don't win by extending your days. You win by not letting the number of your days determine how you live." How do you feel about that idea?

6. What is your "check out time" metaphor? How do you discern when it's time to persist, and when it's time to let go?

Chapter 11 – Walking Her Home as Far as I Could

Summary:

This chapter tenderly recounts Elisa's journey walking alongside her dear friend Diane through the final stages of terminal illness. From the anguish of missed moments to the sacred intimacy of singing Diane into death, the chapter explores presence, denial, spiritual companionship, and the heartbreak of grieving alone. As Elisa navigates hospitals, hospice, and the emotional wilderness of loss, she reflects on her own early grief, the painful echo of being unseen, and the redemptive power of bearing witness. It is a love letter to friendship, a meditation on death, and an offering of holy accompaniment through darkness.

Discussion Questions:

1. Have you ever accompanied someone through the end of their life? What emotions or memories did this chapter stir in you?

2. What does it mean to "walk someone home" spiritually, emotionally, or physically? Have you ever done so?

3. How did Elisa's presence and music become a form of sacred service? Have you ever offered or received that kind of care?

4. Which moments in this chapter felt most sacred or meaningful to you, and why?

5. How did Elisa's childhood grief shape her response to Diane's dying? Can you see echoes of past grief in your present self?

6. What does this chapter teach about the power of presence, even when there are no words to fix the pain?

Chapter 12 – Again!

Summary:

This chapter is a love song to aliveness. *Again* is not a groan, but a gleeful exclamation—a childlike cheer for the wonder of waking up, of being here. Elisa reflects on how the nearness of death sharpened Diane's desire to live—not just to endure, but to savor. Just as ee cummings writes in his poem, everything about the gay great happening illimitably earth is an invitation to say, *Again!* The chapter celebrates this holy appetite for life, the kind that returns not with weariness, but with open arms and a resounding yes.

Discussion Questions:

1. How do you personally respond to the idea that "time is just another word for life"? What does that change, if anything, about how you view your daily routines?

2. Have you ever felt pulled toward darkness or melancholy as part of your identity, like Elisa describes as an Enneagram Four? What helps you shift?

3. Do you relate to the concept of "killing time"? What are some healthier ways you could begin to "redeem the time" in your own life?

4. How do you respond to the chapter's encouragement to rewire the brain through intentional focus? Have you tried practices like gratitude, mindfulness, or savoring?

5. What would it mean for you to wake up tomorrow morning and, like Diane, greet life with the cry, "Again!"? What's one way you could embody that?

Chapter 13 – Shipwrecked

Summary:

In this chapter, Elisa explores the emotional wreckage following the death of a beloved friend, Diane. Through reflections on sacred caregiving, spiritual abandonment, and profound isolation, the chapter examines the toll of cumulative grief. The American denial of death, lack of caregiver support, and unprocessed childhood trauma compound the loss. A visceral, symbolic story of burying a dead kitten in Korea reveals how even small griefs can awaken buried sorrow. By the end, the narrator realizes that healing requires facing not only one loss but a lifelong storm of grief, going back to a forgotten mother wound from early childhood.

Discussion Questions:

1. Have you ever experienced a time in your life that felt like a

shipwreck—where everything familiar or safe was lost? What helped you stay afloat?

2. How do you relate to the idea of cumulative grief—grief layered over time, rather than from a single loss?

3. When, if ever, have you felt like no one had the "script" for what you were going through? What helped you write your own?

4. The narrator describes a culture that avoids talking about death. How has your family or community shaped your view of dying?

5. Can you think of a time when a small or symbolic loss (like the kitten) triggered a flood of older, deeper grief?

6. What does the phrase "At least she knew love" mean to you? Who or what in your life needs that kind of tenderness now?

Chapter 14 – The Vault that Would Not Stay Shut
Summary:

This chapter explores the intense grief Elisa experienced over Diane's death, a loss that unearthed older, unhealed trauma from her childhood—specifically, the death of her brother Brian and the resulting "mother wound." Elisa recounts the bewilderment of others at her prolonged mourning, linking it to a lifetime of feeling abandoned and emotionally starved. Through academic work, especially her dissertation, and eventually trauma therapy, she begins to uncover how dissociation masked decades of unresolved pain. The chapter traces her path from denial to recognition, revealing how Diane's death became the catalyst for confronting—and finally grieving—her deepest wounds.

Discussion Questions:

1. Have you ever been surprised by the depth of your grief over someone who wasn't a close family member? Why do you think certain losses hit harder than others?

2. What relationships in your life have offered you unconditional love or acceptance, as Diane did for Elisa?

3. Have you ever recognized a "script" or pattern in your relationships, as Elisa did with abandonment?

4. How does dissociation—telling a story without feeling—show up in your own life or in others you know?

5. Elisa jokes about writing a dissertation as an "exercise in exorcism." What personal projects in your life have unexpectedly unearthed deep emotions?

6. If you could write a "post-it note" to your younger self about one of your deepest wounds, what would it say?

Chapter 15 – The Mother Wound (Last Day of My Childhood)

Summary:

In this raw and devastating chapter, Elisa recounts the Halloween tragedy that took her younger brother Brian's life and shattered her childhood. Blinded by a costume mask and deaf in one ear, she was unable to grab his hand in time. The trauma was compounded by family silence, parental mental illness, and emotional neglect, resulting in a lifelong "mother wound" and internalized guilt. Through trauma therapy, dissociation began to crack open, revealing buried grief, distorted beliefs about love and worthiness, and suppressed pain. With time, tenderness, and truth-telling, Elisa began to rewrite the script of her life—and reclaim her wholeness.

Discussion Questions:

1. Have you ever blamed yourself for something that happened in your early life? Looking back, can you see that event through a more compassionate lens now?

2. What beliefs about love or worthiness did you absorb in childhood? Are those beliefs still serving you—or are they asking to be re-examined?

3. Has a later loss in your life ever reactivated a much earlier, unprocessed wound? How did you respond? What surprised you about your reaction?

4. How do you typically respond to grief—by expressing, suppressing, or detaching? Where do you think that pattern began?

5. Are there memories you tell like a news report—flat, emotionless, matter-of-fact? What might those stories be protecting you from feeling?

6. What would it mean to you to rewrite a painful memory with greater understanding and truth? How might your relationship with yourself shift?

Chapter 16 – Free Hand-Me-Down Epiphanies, Lightly Used

Summary:

In this chapter, Elisa reflects on the layered healing process that unfolded through trauma therapy, storytelling, and radical self-compassion. As she revisited the story of her brother Brian's death, she unearthed long-buried grief, false guilt, and a mother wound formed in silence. Each retelling brought new epiphanies: children can't grieve developmentally, grieving parents often withdraw, trauma masquerades as toughness, and healing comes slowly—but it comes. From symbolic rituals to anniversary awareness, Elisa reclaims her wholeness verse by verse, like the song she wrote for Brian. Her grief becomes a melody of memory and love—offered freely now, as hand-me-down epiphanies for others.

Discussion Questions:

1. Is there a painful story from your past that you've told so many times it feels flat or scripted? What would happen if you allowed yourself to feel it again with new eyes?

2. Have you mistaken numbness or detachment for strength? What are the signs that it might actually be unresolved grief?

3. When has someone else's silence—especially a parent or caregiver—felt like rejection? Could it have been their way of surviving pain?

4. Have you ever experienced grief from one event unlocking grief

from an earlier one? What did that reveal about your inner world?

5. Do you notice emotional patterns or low points that return around the same time each year? What anniversaries might your soul be tracking?

6. Have you ever found healing by speaking about something your family never discussed? What changed after it was finally named?

Chapter 17 – Refugee from a Boneless Chicken Ranch Rising

Summary:

This chapter traces the long, nonlinear arc of healing after trauma, grief, and emotional collapse. In the wake of deep losses and stalled academic promise, Elisa enters a period of disconnection, humorously likened to a "refugee from a boneless chicken ranch." Through years of geographic wandering, professional limbo, and intense introspection, she slowly reclaims joy, identity, and purpose. Anchored by chosen family, spiritual practice, teaching, and community, her resurrection unfolds not as a miracle but as a gradual reassembly. The chapter offers a hopeful witness: healing is possible—even for those who've felt limp, lost, and completely undone.

Discussion Questions:

1. Elisa's healing took years. How does that challenge or affirm your own expectations about recovery or transformation? Do you think, having seen the components of her healing, that you might be able to heal faster from similar losses?

2. What role has chosen family or unexpected community played in your healing journey?

3. In what ways can joy and grief coexist in your story? How do you recognize both without denying either?

4. Elisa credits her healing not to sudden miracles, but to cumulative choices. Can you name one small choice you've made that has contributed to your long-term growth?

5. What does "resurrection" mean to you—not in a religious sense, but in terms of personal reinvention or reclamation?

6. What do you need right now to begin (or continue) your own rising—from burnout, grief, or a time of emotional collapse?

Chapter 18 – Retelling, Reframing, Rewiring

Summary:

This chapter explores how retelling one's story can rewire the brain and become a path to deep healing after trauma. Drawing on personal grief, trauma therapy, and neuroplasticity, Elisa reframes suffering not as redemptive in itself, but as fertile ground for growth. Through humor, agency, and spiritual reflection, she shows how narrative can transform pain into purpose. Cultural parables, personal poetry, and academic insight weave together to illustrate the power of storytelling in reclaiming identity. Ultimately, this chapter argues that when we consciously reshape our stories, we regain authorship over our lives—even in the shadow of death or disease.

Discussion Questions:

1. What role does storytelling play in your healing or growth journey? Do you find power in retelling your own narrative?

2. Have you ever experienced post-traumatic growth? If so, what did it look like—and what made it possible?

3. How do you respond when someone tells you, "Everything happens for a reason"? Do you agree, disagree, or something in between?

4. Do you relate to the metaphor of "falling in a hole" after loss or trauma? What helped—or might help—you find a door at the bottom?

5. What cultural or family messages have you received about suffering and resilience? How have they shaped the way you grieve or heal?

6. The chapter critiques passive acceptance ("shoganai" / "it is what it is") and champions agency. Where in your life are you reclaiming agency right now?

Chapter 19 – DIY Resurrection: The Tools I Used to Reclaim My Life

Summary:

In this chapter, Elisa reflects on how she emerged from the depths of grief not through a grand plan but by slowly discovering—and later naming—ten essential tools that fueled her resurrection. After years of failed strategies like isolation, busyness, and longing for the "old self," she found healing through trauma-informed therapy, community, spirituality, mindset transformation, intentional gratitude, goal setting, service, and creativity. These weren't magic steps, but small, daily choices that slowly rewired her mind and soul. Now, she offers these hand-me-down epiphanies to others, reminding us that we, too, have tools in our metaphorical junk drawers—and can begin again.

1. What strategies have you used to survive pain that, in hindsight, didn't actually help you heal? How can you show yourself compassion for trying?

2. Which parts of your story do you keep trying to "go back to," and what might happen if you chose to move forward instead?

3. What tools are already in your "kitchen drawer"—those internal or accessible resources you've forgotten you have?

4. What's one small spiritual or grounding practice that helps you feel connected to something bigger than your pain?

5. What is something only *you* can give to others, even in your brokenness? How might sharing it bring healing to both of you?

6. What form of creativity brings you joy—and when's the last time you gave yourself permission to fully enter that flow?

Chapter 20 – Taking Cancer's Keys

Summary:

In this chapter, Elisa describes the moment she was diagnosed with Stage IV pancreatic cancer—not as a collapse into despair, but as a battle cry to reclaim authorship over her story. Drawing from the grief and growth she experienced after Diane's death, she refuses to let cancer define her narrative. Instead, she identifies seven keys she took back: light, love, purpose, gratitude, humor, intentional relationships, and reframing. With boldness, wit, and soul, she models how to meet death without surrendering to it—choosing joy, teaching others to grieve well, and leaving love behind as her final, living legacy.

Discussion Questions:

1. When have you mistaken having no control over an event for having no control over your *response* to it? What's one small way you could reclaim agency now?

2. Who or what has prepared you—intentionally or unintentionally—for challenges you've faced? How can their story or wisdom continue to shape your own?

3. What's one act of love or healing you could offer—even in the middle of your own struggle? How might that become part of your legacy?

4. If you had just a short time left, what would you want to say to the people closest to you? What gift—tangible or intangible—would you want to leave behind?

5. How has humor served you in times of deep pain or fear? Can you think of a moment when laughter helped shift your perspective?

6. Which of the seven keys (light, love, purpose, gratitude, humor, relational closure, reframing) resonates most with you right now? How could you begin using it today?

Chapter 21 – Having a Little Chat with Bob (and Then My Peeps)

Summary:

This chapter explores the common misinterpretations of Kübler-Ross's five stages of grief and reframes them through Elisa's lived experience with terminal illness. With wit and candor, Elisa unpacks her reaction to a death sentence—not with anger or denial, but with bemused indignation, acceptance, and logistical precision. She reflects on her lack of fear, the cultural myths about grief and dying, and the absurdity of timing: finally healed, finally joyful—and now dying. Through reflections, dark humor, and fierce love for her people, she begins to make peace with the absurd and sacred task of preparing to die well.

Discussion Questions:

1. How did this chapter challenge or expand your understanding of Kübler-Ross's five stages of grief? Did anything surprise you about how the stages were originally intended?

2. Elisa writes about not feeling anger or denial. Have you ever experienced grief or trauma without those stages? What did it look like for you?

3. How do you relate to the idea of preparing for death like planning a wedding? What kinds of emotional or logistical preparation do you think are most important?

4. Elisa says, "Your soul keeps track," referring to anniversaries of loss. Have you ever experienced unexpected grief or emotions around certain dates?

5. How did Elisa's reflections on her mother's grief shift your perspective on generational loss or resilience?

6. What do you think it means to "survive death," as Elisa puts it? Can legacy, memory, or love offer a kind of survival?

Chapter 22 – The Joy of Loving Me

Summary:

This chapter honors the deep love, reciprocity, and soul-level caregiving that surrounded Elisa during her cancer journey. Drawing on lifelong reflections on interdependence, disability, and dignity, she affirms the sacredness of chosen family, emotional agency, and mutual service. With humor and fierce clarity, she outlines her caregiving philosophy, insisting on dignity, self-expression, and contribution even in decline. From practical end-of-life logistics to her wish to remain emotionally present and respected, she offers a powerful testament to the joy of being truly loved—and the equal joy of loving others with intentionality, clarity, and grace.

Discussion Questions:

1. How do you define dignity in caregiving—both giving and receiving it?

2. Have you ever had trouble accepting help? What made it hard, and what helped you let go (or not)?

3. What role has chosen family played in your life? Who are the "siblings of your soul"?

4. What unspoken caregiving philosophies or expectations exist in your family or culture? How do they affect you?

5. How do you balance your need for independence with your need for connection and support?

6. What kind of end-of-life experience do you hope for? Have you shared those hopes with anyone?

Chapter 23 – Why Me?

Summary:

In this deeply philosophical chapter, Elisa reflects on the futility—and occasional utility—of asking "Why?" in the face of suffering. Drawing from personal experience, spiritual traditions, and thinkers like Viktor Frankl and Nietzsche, she dismantles the idea that suffering must come with a cosmic explanation. Instead, she champions the power of meaning-making: our ability to assign purpose to even the darkest chapters of our lives. Whether through faith, humor, or resilience, we can transform pain into beauty, not by knowing why, but by deciding what to do with what we're given—and how to live with courage, creativity, and love.

Discussion Questions:

1. When in your life have you asked "Why me?"—and what did you hope the answer would give you?

2. Do you resonate more with the need for meaning or the need for control when facing suffering? Why?

3. How does the idea that "you get to decide the meaning" challenge or empower you?

4. Have you ever reframed a painful experience into something redemptive or beautiful? What helped you do that?

5. Is there a time you were comforted—or hurt—by someone saying, "Everything happens for a reason"? How do you interpret that phrase now?

6. What's your "why"—the reason you go on, the force that animates your story? Has it changed over time?

Chapter 24 – Why I Am Not Afraid to Die

Summary:

This chapter explores the evolution of Elisa's relationship with death—from childhood trauma to terminal diagnosis. Through reflections on aging, loss, and the illusions of control and entitlement, she arrives at a startling peace. Death, once a terrifying stalker, becomes a familiar companion. The chapter challenges cultural denial of mortality, questions of "why me," and affirms the freedom to make meaning out of suffering. With humor, grit, and poetic clarity, Elisa reminds us that there are fates worse than death—and that life, with all its texture and beauty, is a miracle worth savoring until the final breath.

Discussion Questions:

1. What emotions arise when you think about your own death? How have those feelings changed over time?

2. Have you ever experienced a moment when death felt close—either your own or someone else's? How did it shape your view of life?

3. Do you believe there are fates worse than death? If so, what are they for you?

4. What does a "life well lived" mean to you? Are you on the path toward that vision?

5. Have you ever assigned meaning to your suffering? If so, how has that reframed your experience?

6. How do you respond to platitudes like "everything happens for a reason"? What meaning would you rather claim for your life's hardest moments?

7. If you had one year left, what would you stop doing—and what would you begin? Why wait?

Chapter 25 – The Much-Maligned Shadow of Death

Summary:

This chapter invites readers to reimagine death not as a dark menace but as a sacred companion that enhances life's beauty. Drawing from scripture, Rumi, and lived experience, it explores the paradox that joy and suffering are interwoven and that the antidote to pain is often hidden within it. Elisa reflects on trauma, healing, and the technicolor holiness of brokenness transfigured by love. Death is not the enemy of life—it is its sharpest revealer. When we stop running from grief and mortality, we begin to savor the miracle of now and live with radical aliveness, wonder, and gratitude.

Elisa reframes death and grief not as a monster, but as a misunderstood companion—a shadow that, when acknowledged, illuminates life in technicolor. Drawing from mysticism, scripture, and her own experience, she shows how befriending death can awaken gratitude, clarity, and fierce joy. This chapter invites the reader to stop running from mortality and instead turn toward it with curiosity, courage, and a sense of sacred wonder.

Discussion Questions:

1. How has your relationship to the idea of death changed over time, if at all?

2. What are the "technicolor" moments in your life that you only noticed because of a shadow?

3. What pain in your past, if any, has made you more capable of joy or compassion?

4. When you think of your own mortality, what emotions arise—and what do they teach you about how you're living now?

5. Can you identify a moment when suffering gave you strength or insight you didn't know you had?

6. If you were to die tomorrow, what would you most want your loved ones to remember—not about your death, but your way of being alive?

Chapter 26 – Life Is Not Beautiful Because It Is Long

Summary:

This chapter is a luminous meditation on mortality, presence, and joy. Drawing from personal experiences of loss, diagnosis, and spiritual awakening, the narrator explores how life's brevity makes it more precious—not less. From savoring everyday pleasures like brushing teeth or smelling peonies, to embracing the full range of human emotion, even rage, the essay celebrates life's technicolor vibrancy. Grief and joy are revealed as partners, not opposites, and meaning arises from fully inhabiting each moment. Life is not beautiful because it lasts, but because we live it deeply—awake, astonished, and grateful for every fleeting breath.

Discussion Questions:

1. How has your relationship with time changed after experiencing loss, illness, or another major life disruption?

2. Have you ever dismissed something as "pointless" that later revealed itself to be deeply nourishing or essential?

3. How do you think grief and joy can coexist in your life? Can you recall a moment when they did?

4. What are the "peonies" in your life—the fleeting pleasures you forget to savor?

5. What does it mean to you to live in technicolor? What practices might help you cultivate that vivid presence?

6. If you knew your life was short, what would you stop doing? What would you start doing with more intention?

Chapter 27 – Metaphors I Live By

Summary:

This chapter explores how the language we use—especially metaphors—shapes our understanding of illness, identity, and healing. Drawing on linguistic relativity, Elisa questions war metaphors commonly used to describe cancer, favoring more compassionate and collaborative images like cleansing or transformation. She reflects on cancer not only as disease but as metaphor: a force that exposes what's hidden, rekindles lost relationships, and clarifies what matters most. With honesty and nuance, the chapter affirms that suffering can be a catalyst for growth—not by force, but by reframing, reclaiming language, and honoring our sacred agency in narrating our own lives.

Discussion Questions:

1. What metaphors have you inherited or used to describe your own struggles—illness, grief, or otherwise? How have they shaped your experience?

2. How do you feel about the common war metaphors surrounding cancer (e.g., "battle," "fight," "survivor")? Do they empower you, burden you, or something else?

3. Can you recall a time when the language others used about your

situation affected your emotional response—for better or worse?

4. If you were to create a metaphor that better fits your personal healing journey, what might it be?

5. Elisa speaks of cancer as a "spiritual CT scan." What might a scan of your soul reveal at this moment?

6. The chapter ends with the idea of "sacred agency." What does that phrase mean to you? Where do you feel agency in your life story right now?

Chapter 28 – Hope Management

Summary:

"Hope Management" explores how individuals navigate uncertainty in the face of serious illness, especially cancer. Drawing on personal experience and the story of a friend, Elisa challenges the "battle" metaphor and argues for a more nuanced, patient-led philosophy of hope. The chapter emphasizes the importance of knowing your preferences around medical information, preparing emotionally and practically for all outcomes, and choosing hope intentionally—not blindly. With humor, clarity, and compassion, Elisa invites readers to reflect on mortality, embrace uncertainty, and design a beautiful, meaningful life—and death—guided by honesty, agency, and love.

Discussion Questions:

1. How do you typically respond to uncertainty—do you seek clarity and control, or try to stay present without knowing outcomes?

2. Have you ever communicated your preferences around difficult news or medical information? How might doing so empower you?

3. When have you experienced a moment that felt like a spiritual "CT scan"—something that revealed what was really going on inside?

4. How do you personally define hope? Is it a feeling, a choice, a

strategy, or something else?

5. What role does cultural messaging (like American optimism or the "fight" mentality) play in your attitudes toward illness or death?

6. When has false positivity—or someone else's version of "staying strong"—left you feeling unseen or unsupported?

7. What would it mean for you to "make your dying a work of art"?

8. If you could offer one lasting emotional or spiritual gift to those you love, what would it be—and are you preparing it now?

Chapter 29 – Gifts of a Death Sentence

Summary:

After a shocking misdiagnosis of terminal pancreatic cancer, Elisa discovers she has a treatable lymphoma instead—an unexpected reprieve that becomes a profound spiritual awakening. She reflects on the intense clarity, restored relationships, and deep gratitude that emerged in the shadow of death. Cancer became a lens that revealed her courage, inner peace, and the soul-deep wealth of love in her life. Rather than feeling angry about the error, she sees the misdiagnosis as a sacred gift—one that shifted her relationship to time, possessions, purpose, and people. In her words: "I would absolutely order again."

Discussion Questions:

1. Have you ever experienced a moment that radically shifted your view of life, like Elisa's misdiagnosis did for her? What changed for you?

2. How does the idea of seeing cancer—or any hardship—as a "gift" sit with you? What gifts, if any, have come from your own struggles?

3. Elisa talks about discovering she wasn't afraid of death. What do you imagine your reaction might be if faced with a terminal diagnosis?

4. How might your relationships change if you truly believed your time was limited? Who would you reach out to?

5. Elisa redefined success by focusing on love and soul nourishment over money or status. How do you define a successful life?

6. She says "every day is a special occasion." What would shift for you if you fully embraced that mindset?

Chapter 30 – More Than a Happy Ending

Summary:

In this closing reflection, Elisa compares the emotional healing journey to a slow, nourishing resurrection—one that doesn't have a clear endpoint or bell to ring. Unlike chemotherapy's celebratory finish, soul healing unfolds gradually, often invisibly, through daily choices and quiet courage. She recounts the "superfood" ingredients that saved her life: trauma therapy, community, spiritual practice, gratitude, creativity, and more. From blob to blossom, her journey became a slow-becoming rather than a sudden transformation. She encourages readers to begin wherever they are—with one breath, one book, or one kind act—and reminds us that our unique healing journeys feed not just ourselves, but the world.

Discussion Questions:

1. What moment in your life might have deserved a bell—even if no one else saw it as a triumph? How might you honor it now?

2. Are you in a "blob" phase of your life right now—or emerging into something new? What's one gentle next step you feel ready for?

3. Is there a part of your healing journey you've discounted because it didn't come with a dramatic transformation? What would it mean to honor that slow progress?

4. Which of the ten "superfood" tools resonated most with you? Is there one you feel ready to explore or return to?

5. What small act of kindness—toward yourself or someone

else—might become a seed for resurrection today?

6. Have you been waiting to "feel ready" before beginning to heal, create, or love again? What if readiness isn't a feeling but a choice?

Epilogue
Summary:

In the epilogue, Elisa reflects on surviving cancer after a terminal misdiagnosis, celebrating her remission and eventual declaration of being "cured." She affirms that cancer didn't awaken her—it confirmed a healing journey already underway. By the time of her diagnosis, she had made peace with death, found joy in life's small pleasures, and embraced resurrection after earlier grief. Cancer, she writes, wasn't a crucible but a proof of life. With grace, gratitude, and humor, she urges readers to do the hard work of healing, not to wait for crisis, and to wake up fully before they die.

Discussion Questions:

1. What does the phrase "I tested positive—for life" mean to you personally?

2. Have you ever experienced a moment that felt like a "proof of life"? What was it?

3. Elisa distinguishes between healing over time and healing with intention. What intentional steps have you taken—or could you take—toward your own healing?

4. How do you respond to the idea that "life is not beautiful because it is long...but because it is deep"?

5. What parts of your story would you want to be complete before your own life ends?

6. How has grief shaped your understanding of love and joy?

7. Elisa says she was "already awake" when cancer came. What does being "awake" mean to you?

8. Do you believe suffering can confirm healing rather than break you further? Why or why not?

9. How might it change your life to live with the awareness that "we all have a terminal diagnosis"?

10. What would "waking before you die" look like in your own life right now?

If you've made it all the way here — through the shadows, the snacks, the songs, and the questions —I hope you know you're not walking alone. Take good care of your beautiful, light-loving heart. See you out there.

Late Night Snacks for the Soul: A Charcuterie Board of Light

Notes on Quotes

S o many questions emerge in the Shadow.

If the answers are "blowing in the wind," I believe that wind is the breath of the divine Spirit as it flows through the hearts and minds of many luminaries from across time and around the world. The voices that have spoken healing and peace to me harken from as long ago as the book of Job to the present day. The voices come from the hearts and minds of poets, mystics, philosophers, academics and other writers.

Perhaps it is cliché to say that I stand on the shoulders of giants, but my voice is certainly a confluence of other voices—with a nod to Bakhtin I would build on his idea of dialogism and call it interdialogicality, all these dialogues intersecting, all these deep conversations cross-pollinating as it were.

I would urge you not to stop with my words, but to go and hunt down some of these other voices to maintain a steady diet of spiritual nourishment.

These quotes have been used in accordance with fair use principles. I often imagine sitting in a room with all of those who spoke them—an anteroom of heaven, filled with luminous conversation. Below are some of the revered voices whose words echo through these pages.

Have what you're hungry for; put the rest back in the fridge for later.

- **James Allen** – a British philosophical writer best known for his 1903 work *As a Man Thinketh*, a cornerstone in the self-help and New Thought movements. Allen famously asserted, "Circumstances don't make the man. They reveal him." In this memoir, I gently revise that claim: I believe that circumstances both reveal and shape us—but the shaping is not automatic; it is under our conscious direction. Allen's central idea—that our inner life is powerful and formative—resonates deeply here, not as a simplistic promise of mind-over-matter, but as an invitation to agency. When life exposes our vulnerabilities, it also offers us a mirror, not to shame us, but to help us clarify who we are becoming. In that sense, Allen's legacy affirms a central theme of this book: that we can work with what life gives us, and that reflection, narrative, and intention are tools for transformation.

- **The Apostle Paul** – Elisa quotes his words, *"I rejoice in my suffering,"* because they reflect the radical alchemy of spiritual transformation, turning pain into purpose. Paul's letters frame suffering not as punishment or evidence of divine absence, but as a crucible for growth and grace. In Romans 5:3, he writes: *"Not only so, but we also glory in our sufferings, because we know that suffering produces perseverance."* And in Colossians 1:24: *"I am now rejoicing in my sufferings for your sake..."* These verses became quiet companions during treatment—not as prescriptions, but as possibilities.

- **Brené Brown** – Researcher and author of *The Gifts of Imperfection* and *Atlas of the Heart* (among so many other brilliant books), quoted for her insight that hope is learned. Her work on vulnerability and emotional resilience are deeply resonant with Elisa's understanding of courage, healing, and the role of faith in overcoming trauma.

- **Brendon Burchard** – Elisa quotes his daily reflection—*"Did I live? Did I love? Did I matter?"*—because it resonates so deeply with what she hoped to leave behind. Facing death, these became her core questions too. Not whether she was successful, but whether she was meaningful in the lives of others.

- **Marc Chagall** – Elisa quotes his line, *"Art must be an expression of love, or it is nothing,"* because it encapsulates the driving force behind this memoir. She never set out to write a medical record or a textbook on grief—she set out to make beauty from brokenness, to love people through language. Like Chagall's luminous, dreamlike paintings, her hope is that this book glows with the colors of emotion, memory, and soul.

- **Pema Chödrön** – Elisa recommends *When Things Fall Apart* because the author's voice is like a hand resting gently on your back during free fall. Her Buddhist wisdom does not rush to fix or explain pain—it invites us to stay with it, breathe through it, and find our center even in the storm.

- **Leonard Cohen** – "There is a crack in everything, that's how the light gets in." Leonard Cohen, deeply influenced by Jewish mysticism and the Kabbalistic tradition, gave us this now-iconic line in his song *Anthem*. The image of brokenness as a vessel for divine light is rooted in the Kabbalistic idea of *sheviratha-kelim*—the shattering of vessels that made space for divine sparks to scatter throughout the world. Healing, then, is not a return to perfection but a gathering of scattered light through our cracks. I hear in Cohen's words the same sacred echo as Rumi's: "The wound is the place where the Light enters you." Both mystics invite us to stop hiding our wounds and begin honoring them as doorways to wholeness. My life, too, has taught me: the cracks weren't the failure. They were the invitation.

- **Mihaly Csikszentmihalyi** – Best known for his research on flow states, argues that creativity is not merely about artistic talent or innovation—it is a profound source of human fulfillment. In *Creativity: Flow and the Psychology of Discovery and Invention*, he suggests that engaging in creative work immerses us in moments of deep focus, purpose, and joy. These "flow states"—where time seems to disappear and self-consciousness fades—are among the most satisfying experiences we can have. Creativity, in this sense, is not a luxury or a personality trait; it is a psychological nourishment, a way to feel alive, connected, and meaningful. For those of us grieving or rebuilding our lives after trauma, creativity becomes not just a tool of self-expression but a lifeline to wholeness.

- **E.E. Cummings** – Poet, quoted in full for *"i thank you god for most this amazing day,"* a poem recited in one of the memoir's most sacred moments. His ecstatic reverence for life resonated with both Elisa and her beloved Diane.

- **Charles Dickens – "Recalled to life."** In *A Tale of Two Cities*, this phrase is first used to describe the resurrection-like return of Dr. Manette, who has been freed after eighteen years of unjust imprisonment. Dickens uses it to evoke the shock, disorientation, and slow reentry into life after a long period of darkness. Elisa adopts this language to describe her own emergence from the emotional catacombs of grief and trauma—a slow, soul-deep transformation that felt less like recovery and more like resurrection. Her healing was not a return to her old self, but a reclamation of life from the shadow of death.

- **Annie Dillard** – Dillard's prose is fierce and luminous. Her books *Holy the Firm* and *For the Time Being* taught Elisa that beauty and terror are twin flames in the human experience. Dillard writes with the eyes of a mystic and the pen of a poet—she gave Elisa permission to ask unanswerable questions and still keep writing.

- **Norman Doidge** – In *The Brain That Changes Itself*, psychiatrist and researcher Norman Doidge explores the revolutionary science of neuroplasticity—the brain's ability to rewire itself throughout life. Through powerful case studies, Doidge shows that healing is not   limited by age or past trauma; instead, the mind can adapt, recover, and even transform. Elisa draws on this understanding when she describes the slow but real rewiring of her trauma-scarred brain. Her memoir echoes Doidge's hopeful premise: that deliberate practice, reframing, and compassionate attention can literally reshape our inner landscape. The book lends scientific grounding to her lived experience of healing through choice and presence.

- **Mary Douglas** – Anthropologist Mary Douglas famously defined dirt as "matter out of place"—not just filth, but disorder. Many cultures respond to that disorder with rituals of cleansing, aimed at the body, the soul, or both. Elisa refers to this idea in her urge to "wash" cancer out of her body, as something out of order as opposed to using a martial metaphor.

- **Glennon Doyle** – Memoirist, activist, and truth-teller extraordinaire. Elisa quotes her admonition, *"Do not disappoint yourself,"* because it cracked something open in her. Glennon reminds us that self-betrayal is the deepest cut, and that self-trust is the first act of courage. Her writing feels like a handheld out across the abyss. Elisa hopes one day to thank her in person—with tears and laughter and maybe a shared plate of fried mushrooms.

- **Ecclesiastes** – Elisa sympathized with Solomon—Israel's golden king—writing in his despondency, *"All is futility and a striving after wind."* He had "everything," but the epiphany is when the soul realizes that none of the "everything" was ever the thing.

- **Robert A. Emmons** – In *Thanks!*, Emmons—one of the leading researchers on gratitude—demonstrates that regularly practicing gratitude significantly boosts happiness and physical health. His findings suggest that even simple acts like keeping a gratitude journal can reduce depression, improve sleep, and strengthen relationships. I found his research not only affirming, but galvanizing. Gratitude became one of the keystones in my healing—not because it erased suffering, but because it helped me honor what remained, what grew, what glowed in the dark. Emmons shows that gratitude isn't naïve—it's brave, disciplined, and transformative.

- **Enneagram** – The Enneagram is a dynamic personality framework that maps nine core types, each representing a distinct way of seeing and engaging with the world. Rooted in ancient spiritual traditions and modern psychology, it's often used as a tool for self-awareness, growth, and compassion. Rather than putting people in rigid boxes, the Enneagram invites curiosity about our motivations, fears, and desires. It helps illuminate both our gifts and our automatic patterns, encouraging transformation through conscious awareness. At its best, the Enneagram is not about ego reinforcement but about soul work—returning to our truest self beyond the masks we wear.

- **Bruce Feiler** – Coined the term *lifequake* to describe a major, identity-shaking disruption—like illness, loss, or upheaval—that forces   profound personal transformation. In *Life Is in the Transitions*, he outlines how we move through these events in phases: the Long Goodbye, the Messy Middle, and the New Beginning. Elisa was introduced to this term by Saleema Vellani through her book *Innovation Starts With I*, which explores how self-discovery and resilience fuel innovation. The word *lifequake* gave Elisa language for the seismic shifts her own life had undergone—and a framework for understanding how to reassemble identity after everything falls apart.

- **Kathleen Ferrara** – In *Therapeutic Ways with Words*, linguistic scholar Kathleen Ferrara explores how talk therapy functions not just as emotional support but as a distinct genre of discourse with its own rituals, roles, and transformative power. Drawing from real therapy transcripts, she shows how language—carefully shaped and relationally offered—can construct new realities, reframe identities, and facilitate healing. Elisa's memoir echoes Ferrara's insights by demonstrating how the very act of retelling and reframing one's story, especially in the presence of a trusted therapist, can rewire thought patterns and open paths to transformation. Language doesn't just reflect healing—it enacts it.

- **Viktor Frankl** – Holocaust survivor and author of *Man's Search for Meaning*, quoted for his belief in the redemptive power of human choice and the enduring freedom to find meaning in suffering. His work profoundly resonated with Elisa's reflections on agency, identity, and the art of living with intention even in the face of death.

- **Barbara Fredrickson** – In *Positivity*, psychologist Barbara Fredrickson doesn't argue for shallow optimism but for a scientifically grounded shift in perspective. Her "broaden-and-build" theory demonstrates that positive emotions like joy, gratitude, serenity, and hope don't just feel good—they expand our awareness, increase resilience, and help us build enduring resources for life. Elisa draws from Fredrickson's work to show how positivity was not a denial of her suffering, but a choice to see beauty, to reframe, and to allow glimmers of light even in the shadow of death. Fredrickson's research affirms that cultivating small moments of positive emotion isn't a betrayal of grief, but a vital tool for emotional healing and long-term transformation.

- **Robert Frost** – America's poet, quoted here for his line, *"The best way out is always through,"* which has become a kind of spiritual axiom for Elisa. But her love for Frost runs far deeper than this single line. His poems—memorized, recited, and lived—have shaped her voice and her vision. Whether walking through woods on a snowy evening or standing at the fork of a yellow road, she's often found herself accompanied by his language, like a companion who knows the path even when she does not.

- **Diana Gabaldon** – Novelist and storyteller extraordinaire, Elisa quotes her from *An Echo in the Bone*—*"All loss is one, and one loss becomes all, a single death is the key to all that bars memory"*—because those words unlocked something in her. Her writing reminds us that grief is not linear or isolated, but layered and ancestral, opening doors we didn't know were shut. Gabaldon has a god-like imagination and a heart to match. Her ability to explore love, time, loss, and resurrection through character and plot is unmatched in the modern fiction Elisa reads. She's her favorite contemporary author of fiction, and if the universe is kind, maybe one day Elisa will get to meet her.

- **Elizabeth Gilbert** – Author of *Eat, Pray, Love* and *Big Magic,* and one of the great contemporary voices on creativity, soul-work, and becoming. Elisa quotes her insight that *"frustration is the process,"* a line that helped her stay grounded through the tangled, looping nature of grief and healing. Her work has been a lighthouse through many storms—gentle, wise, and unafraid to tell the truth about love, longing, failure, and starting again. Elizabeth Gilbert makes Elisa believe in beauty as a spiritual practice and friendship as a sacred art.

- **Richard Gillard** – New Zealand hymnwriter, quoted from *"The Servant Song"* for its lyrical prayer: "Will you let me be your servant, let me be as Christ to you?" His words capture the sacred reciprocity at the heart of caregiving and mutual love. Elisa sang this line (terribly, she says, but with love) at the funeral of her stepfather, Gail, who so beautifully embodied it (and who passed away during the writing of this book).

- **Jonathan Haidt** – In *The Happiness Hypothesis*, Haidt explores how hardship can build resilience, a theme that mirrored my own journey. Elisa quoted him while reflecting on her ability to face stage IV cancer with equanimity—not because she believed suffering was sent to prepare her, but because she recognized its effect. Haidt gave her a lens through which to name her survival: she wasn't lucky or superhuman; she had been trained by life. His work helped her frame her emotional endurance not as accidental, but as earned.

- **Heidi E. Hamilton, Ph.D** – Elisa's dissertation mentor, Dr. Hamilton reminds her—both through her scholarship and her spirit—that language is not only for conveying information but also for connection, healing, and love. Her work with Alzheimer's patients, especially in *Glimmers*, revealed to Elisa the profound presence available even when memory fails. Dr. Hamilton shows that even in circumstances that might seem very grim, there is light if you have eyes to see it. The idea that "mindlessness can be a path to mindfulness" helped shape Elisa's understanding of suffering and presence in the final stages of life. Dr. Hamilton's compassion continues to be a model for how to witness and honor the humanity of others.

- **HarperCollins UK** – A 2024 survey revealed that 29% of 14–25-year-olds strongly identify as readers—and those who read daily are far more likely to describe themselves as "very happy." I love this. It confirms what I've long felt: reading feeds the soul. For young readers especially, books offer not just escape, but identity, meaning, and mental health benefits that go beyond entertainment. Reading is one of the most accessible forms of self-care—and transformation—I know.

- **The Hebrew Bible – Job, Genesis, Ecclesiastes** –Elisa references these ancient texts not for comfort, but for context. The existential anguish of Job, the stark beauty of Genesis, and the philosophical resignation of Ecclesiastes (attributed to Solomon) all helped shape Elisa's own reflections on suffering, mortality, and the hunger for meaning. These are not soothing texts—but they are honest ones, and Elisa wanted that same honesty in her own pages. Moreover, they are classics that must be acknowledged in the literature of grief.

- **William Ernest Henley** – Best known for his poem *Invictus*, Henley's defiant spirit has long spoken to those facing hardship with dignity and determination. Elisa quotes his famous closing lines, *"I am the master of my fate, I am the captain of my soul"*—because they name something fierce and sacred in the human will: the refusal to be entirely undone by suffering. Henley wrote these words from a hospital bed after losing a leg to tuberculosis. Elisa carried them like a mantra through her own resurrection, not because she believed she could control the outcome, but because they reminded her she could still steer her own spirit. His voice joins hers in the quiet resolve to live and love fully no matter what.

- **Ryan Holiday** – Elisa references the title of Holiday's book, *The Obstacle Is the Way*, because it speaks so directly to her experience of post-traumatic growth. What nearly broke her—grief, loss, illness—ultimately became the very path to healing. His stoic reframing of   hardship as the route, not the detour, resonated deeply with her own journey through despair and into light.

- **Oliver Wendell Holmes, Jr.** – Holmes referred to words as the *skins of living thoughts*—a phrase that captures the way language can preserve the vitality of feeling and experience. In this memoir, where words are tasked with carrying the weight of memory, grief, and joy, Holmes reminds Elisa that language is not merely decorative. It is the sacred skin that allows thought to live outside the mind and across time.

- **Arianna Huffington** – *"Stop just assuming you have a full lifetime to do whatever it is you dream of doing."* This quote reminds Elisa that dreams deferred can become dreams discarded. It urges urgency—not panic, but presence. Elisa spent far too many years believing she had time. Time to heal, time to write, time to live as she was meant to. But terminal illness has a way of stripping away illusions. Arianna's words echo what life has already taught Elisa: if something matters to your soul, start now. We are not promised someday. We have this day.

- **John 21:18 (Jesus to Peter)** – "Truly I tell you, when you were young, you dressed yourself, and walked where you wanted to. But when you are old, you will stretch out your hands, and another will dress you, and carry you where you do not want to go." Elisa kept returning to this verse during treatment, when she was at the mercy of so many others—doctors, nurses, scans, side effects. It speaks to the surrender of control that aging and illness demand—and the strange, sacred dignity that can arise in that surrender.

- **Kansas – "Dust in the Wind"** – This iconic 1977 song by the band Kansas opens with the haunting line, *"All we are is dust in the wind,"* and it became the perfect frame for her section on suffering, mortality, and meaning. Growing up in Kansas (one of the epicenters of the Great Dust Bowl), she always felt this lyric carried extra weight—a kind of whispered reminder that everything is fleeting. But she doesn't quote it to express nihilism. Instead, she uses it to enter a deeper conversation about impermanence, presence, and how we make peace with the inevitability of loss. As the song says, *"Nothing lasts forever but the earth and sky,"* and maybe love, too.

- **Elisabeth Kübler-Ross** – Psychiatrist and author of *On Death and Dying*, quoted in Elisa's reflections on the five stages of grief and how her work has been misunderstood and perhaps over extrapolated in popular culture.

- **Harold Kushner** – Rabbi and author of *When Bad Things Happen to Good People*, Kushner's compassionate theology has offered comfort and clarity to countless people facing unimaginable loss. Elisa references his work while reflecting on the human impulse to ask "Why?" in the face of suffering. Kushner doesn't offer easy answers—he offers presence, honesty, and a deeply human understanding of pain.

- **Anne Lamott** – Author of *Traveling Mercies* and *Bird by* Bird (among many other wonderful books), for her fierce humor and spiritual candor and her beautiful metaphor of death as a "significant change of address." Elisa had the extreme pleasure of seeing her and Eve Ensler present together a few years ago for their tour on *Notes on Hope* and *In the Body of the World*. She was deeply impressed by the love emanating from that stage.

- **Ellen Langer** – Langer's reflection, echoing Epictetus, that "events don't cause stress; the views you take of events" do, captures the transformative power of narrative. Her work on mindfulness affirmed for Elisa that our suffering is not simply about what happens to us, but how we interpret and integrate those events into our inner lives. This is one of the great acts of agency—retelling the story in a way that heals rather than harms.

- **David Lewis** – In a now-famous 2009 study at the University of Sussex, cognitive neuropsychologist David Lewis found that reading for just six minutes can reduce stress by up to 68%—more than listening to music, walking, or drinking tea. The study affirmed what many of us know intuitively: a good book can calm the nervous system, slow the heart, and transport us somewhere safer, even if only briefly. Reading, then, becomes more than entertainment—it's a healing practice. I included this finding because it echoes my lived experience: the right words at the right time can shift your whole internal weather system.

- **Abraham Lincoln** – Elisa loves this quote attributed to him, *"I want it said of me by those who knew me best, that I always plucked a thistle and planted a flower where I thought a flower would grow."* Whether or not Lincoln actually said it, the sentiment lives at the heart of this memoir. Elisa, too, wants to be remembered not for what she endured, but for the love and beauty she tried to plant wherever she found sorrow.

- **Sonja Lyubomirsky** – In *The How of Happiness*, psychologist Sonja Lyubomirsky presents decades of research on what truly contributes to sustained well-being—and how much of it lies within our control. She identifies intentional activities, such as practicing gratitude, cultivating optimism, and engaging in spiritual or reflective practices, as powerful levers of change. Elisa references Lyubomirsky's work to affirm that happiness is not just a product of external circumstances but of deliberate habits. The memoir aligns with Lyubomirsky's findings by showing how Elisa's consistent, soul-level choices helped rebuild joy from the ashes of grief. Science, in this case, validates lived wisdom.

- **Melody Moezzi** – Iranian American writer and author of *Haldol and Hyacinths* and *The Rumi Prescription*, quoted both for her translations of Rumi (alongside her father) and for her sharp, humorous reflections on American culture. Her work influenced this memoir's exploration of spiritual insight and cultural absurdity.

- **Friedrich Nietzsche** – Philosopher, quoted for his insight "He who has a why to live can bear almost any how." His thoughts on meaning, suffering, and existential agency helped shape Elisa's reflections on narrative, purpose, and the search for meaning in the face of terminal illness.

- **Gabriele Oettingen** – In *Rethinking Positive Thinking: Inside the New Science of Motivation*, psychologist Gabriele Oettingen challenges the cultural obsession with blind optimism. Her research shows that while fantasizing about positive outcomes can feel good in the moment, it often leads to complacency rather than action. What truly drives success and long-term satisfaction, she argues, is a strategy called *mental contrasting*—imagining a desired future while also honestly confronting the obstacles in the way. This grounded hope, rooted in both vision and realism, fosters motivation, resilience, and ultimately, deeper happiness. For those navigating grief, illness, or transformation, Oettingen's work offers a compassionate nudge toward purposeful action—encouraging us to dream, yes, but also to do the hard, hopeful work of getting there.

- **Georgia O'Keeffe** – O'Keeffe once said, "Nobody sees a flower—really—it is so small it takes time." That's what artists like her offer us: the discipline of attention, the radical act of reverence. In a world where beauty so often goes in one eye and out the other, she reminds us to *linger*—to look long enough for the miracle to appear. O'Keeffe's life and art were deeply intertwined, reflecting a philosophy where personal experience and creative expression are inseparable. "Your life is your art, as well as the thing you call your art." While this exact phrasing is widely attributed to O'Keeffe, its precise origin remains elusive. It encapsulates, however, her belief that art is not confined to the canvas but is a reflection of one's entire being and way of living. O'Keeffe's dedication to authenticity and her seamless integration of life and art serve as a testament to this philosophy. This perspective aligns with the themes of this memoir, emphasizing that every facet of life—especially during times of adversity—can be a form of art. It invites readers to view their own lives as creative expressions, where meaning and beauty can be found in everyday moments.

- **Mary Oliver** – Pulitzer Prize–winning poet, quoted for her iconic line, "What will you do with your one wild and precious life?" Her work deepened Elisa's meditation on attention, gratitude, and the urgency of living while we're alive.

- **Dolly Parton** – Dolly is one of Elisa's revered heroes. She mentions her version of *"Have a Little Talk with Jesus"*—a gospel classic that captures the intimacy, comfort, and honesty of spiritual conversation. Dolly's voice makes the plea feel personal, not performative—a reminder that prayer can be a place of presence, not perfection. *(Featured on her 1999 album "Precious Memories," available on most streaming platforms.)*

- **Cesare Pavese** – An Italian poet, novelist, and translator whose work often wrestled with solitude, memory, and the search for meaning in everyday life. This quote—frequently paraphrased as *"We don't remember days, only moments"*—echoes a deeper reflection from his diaries: "We do not remember days; we remember moments. The richness of life lies in memories we have forgotten," (*The Burning Brand: Diaries 1935–1950*). This insight captures the essence of presence and recollection—that our most vivid memories are not shaped by time's calendar, but by the emotional weight and texture of singular, sacred moments. It fits beautifully with the themes of this memoir: that life's depth is found in its luminous, fleeting flashes. The quote reminds us that we live not in spans, but in sparks—and that healing often begins in the noticing.

- **Stephen G. Post** – In his report "It's Good to Be Good," Post draws from decades of interdisciplinary research to show that helping others doesn't just make the world better—it makes *you* better, too. Acts of compassion and generosity are consistently linked to increased happiness, resilience, and even longevity. His work affirms what many of us sense intuitively: when we step outside ourselves to care for others, we often find ourselves healed in the process. Elisa included Post's work because it backs up with data what so many of us have discovered firsthand—service is not a detour from joy. It's one of its clearest paths.

- ***Psalm 17:8*** – *"Hide me in the shadow of your wings."* In a season when the word "shadow" so often connotes fear or death, Elisa finds comfort in David's prayer: "Keep me as the apple of your eye, hide me in the shadow of your wings." This is not the shadow of despair, but of protection. A maternal, enveloping shadow. A place of refuge. When Elisa's own journey brought her into the shadow of death, she began to wonder: What if the shadow isn't only something to fear—but also something to lean into? Something soft, sheltering, even holy?

- **Rabia al-Basri** – An 8th-century Sufi mystic and poet, Rabia al-Basri lived a life of radical love and uncompromising spiritual devotion. That she was able to leave such a lasting legacy as a Muslim woman in early Islamic society is, to Elisa, astonishing and inspiring. Her refusal to seek God out of fear of hell or hope for heaven—only for love—was revolutionary. Elisa quotes her for her luminous expression of divine longing and surrender. She also writes, *"I carry a torch in one hand and a bucket of water in the other: with these things I am going to set fire to Heaven and put out the flames of Hell so that travelers to God can rip the veils and see the real goal."* Rabia's fierce clarity reminds us that true spirituality is not transactional—it is the undoing of the self in the presence of love. Her voice echoes through the centuries, reminding us that the soul has no gender, and that devotion can be a form of holy resistance.

- **Lindsey Roy** – In her TED Talk *Phantom Life: What Trauma Taught Me About Happiness*, Lindsey Roy offers a disarmingly honest and brilliantly human perspective on the hidden advantages of loss. Elisa admires her deeply for the way she reframes trauma—not to gloss over suffering, but to draw attention to the compassion, clarity, and presence it can evoke. She is funny, humble, and quietly revolutionary. From painting toenails with a prosthetic leg propped on a table to noticing the sweetness of her children's empathy, she reminds us that resilience isn't about pretending things are fine—it's about looking for the light, even if it's only the size of a pinprick.

- **Jalāl ad-Dīn Muhammad Rūmī (Rumi)** – Often referred to by Persians as simply Maulana (the Master), he was a 13th-century Persian mystic, theologian, and poet whose words continue to move hearts across cultures and centuries. Rumi wrote not to impress but to *unveil*—to tear the veil between the soul and the Beloved. His verse is infused with longing, surrender, ecstasy, and the ache of separation that ultimately leads to union. A poet of divine love and inner awakening, Rumi reminds us that grief can be the reed through which God breathes music, and that every wound is a doorway to the sacred. Though often quoted in English via the luminous renderings of Coleman Barks, his essence also lives in translations by Melody Moezzi and her father, as well as so many others. His poetry transcends language, doctrine, and even selfhood—calling the reader to die before they die, to burn away what is false, and to dance toward what is real. For Elisa, Rumi is not just a writer but a guide—a soul-whisperer whose words hold her hand when the world is too heavy, and who points again and again to the mystery at the center of love.

- **William Shakespeare** – Quoted from *Hamlet* for the line "Nothing is good or bad, but thinking makes it so." His insight anchors a reflection on cognitive reframing and personal agency.

- **Wallace Stevens** – Elisa references his phrase *"the human rage for order,"* which he used to describe our deep desire to make sense of chaos through art, poetry, and story. Stevens gives language to the persistent human need to know the reason why things happen as they do. Elisa wishes this book too to be a part of that ordering, to give some relief to those asking why.

- **StrengthsFinder** – This is not a quote so much as a gratitude note to the tool that helped Elisa reframe herself not as broken, but as uniquely gifted. According to *StrengthsFinder*, her top five strengths are Connectedness, Input, Strategic, Learner, and Ideation—and, in hindsight, they show up everywhere in this book. Connectedness is the pulse that runs through these pages: the insistence that no pain is wasted, that grief and love exist in relationship, and that our stories are threads in a larger tapestry. Input shows up in the kaleidoscope of references—spiritual texts, neuroscience, memoir, metaphysics, and pop culture—gathered not to impress but to nourish. Strategic is the reason this book has any arc at all. Even when life felt chaotic, she was crafting a path forward—for herself and, she hopes, for others. Learner explains why she didn't stay in the pit. She read, she listened, she went to therapy, she kept going. And she kept writing. Ideation is what turned the pit into poetry and the grief into metaphor. It's the reason she called that chapter "Refugee from a Boneless Chicken Ranch Rising." This tool didn't just show her who she was; it helped her remember that who she is was never the problem. She just needed to reclaim herself—and write from there.

- **"Talk About Suffering Here Below"** – Elisa references the haunting opening line of this old spiritual: *"Talk about suffering here below..."*—a line that echoes in the hearts of those who've walked through sorrow and come out singing. The song is often passed down through Appalachian and gospel traditions, carried in voices both raw and reverent. Elisa especially loves Phil Keaggy's rendition, which holds the ache and the hope in perfect tension. This line, and the song it belongs to, reminds her that suffering and joy are not opposites—they're companions on the pilgrim path. To talk about suffering here below is, in its way, a sacred act of remembering, testifying, and finding beauty in the wail. It reminds her, further, that there is a sweet communion with the divine in the presence of suffering.

- **Deborah Tannen, Ph. D** – Linguist, memoirist, and master of nuance in everyday talk, (and mentor for the analysis chapters of Elisa's   dissertation), Tannen's work has long shaped how she thinks about conversation as both connection and meaning-making. In *The Argument Culture* she describes how American discourse has become saturated with conflict metaphors—turning every disagreement into a battle, every conversation into a fight. As someone who has lived through literal and metaphorical battles, Elisa has come to believe that not everything needs to be framed as a fight. Sometimes the bravest thing we can do is refuse the war metaphor altogether.

She also quotes Dr. Tannen's memoir *Finding My Father*, where she recounts a moment over pizza when her father, then in his nineties, said: *"I expect one morning to wake up and find myself dead, and I wouldn't mind. I wasn't alive before I was born, and I didn't mind at all."* Elisa just loves that. It's so tender and wry—an almost Buddhist acceptance of mortality, wrapped in fatherly pragmatism. Tannen captures the power of seemingly ordinary dialogue to reveal the deepest truths about who we are, and how we live and die.

- **Dylan Thomas** – Elisa quotes Thomas's line, *"After the first death, there is no other,"* because it captures the way one early loss can echo through a lifetime. For Elisa, that first death was her brother's, and every grief since has been a variation on that original wound.

- **Henry David Thoreau** – Elisa returns often to these well-worn, well-loved words of Henry David Thoreau—words that have echoed in the hearts of seekers for generations. *"I went to the woods because I wished to live deliberately..."* In facing death, Elisa was given the same stripped-down clarity: the desire to confront only the essential facts of life. Not to live what was not life, not to practice resignation unless it was absolutely necessary. Thoreau wanted to suck the marrow from life. She wanted to taste it too—and to know, when she came to die, that she had lived not just deeply, but awake.

- **Eckhart Tolle** – Elisa referenced Tolle's insight that "there is no time *but* the present" from *The Power of Now* to reinforce the memoir's core message of presence and savoring. His teachings on stillness, consciousness, and the now have offered a powerful counterpoint to anxiety and despair—and a grounding framework for joy, even in the shadow of death.

- **Vincent Van Gogh** – The Dutch post-impressionist painter whose tormented inner life gave rise to some of the most beloved and emotionally resonant works of Western art. Though plagued by mental illness, poverty, and rejection in his lifetime, van Gogh's letters reveal a sensitive soul with a fierce love for beauty, humanity, and God. He once wrote, *"I think there is nothing more artistic than loving people,"* a sentiment that transforms love itself into a creative act—one that, like art, demands vulnerability, presence, and soul. In many ways, his life exemplifies the painful tension between suffering and transcendence—between madness and meaning—making him a fitting companion in any reflection on grief, beauty, and the redemptive power of loving anyway.

- **Robert Waldinger and Marc Schulz** – In *The Good Life*, Waldinger and Schulz distill insights from the Harvard Study of Adult   Development, the world's longest scientific study of happiness. Their key finding? The quality of our relationships—more than wealth, career success, or even physical health—predicts long-term well-being. Elisa weaves this insight into her memoir by highlighting the role of chosen family, community, and connection in her resurrection. The book affirms what many intuitively know: love is the lifeblood of healing. In moments of despair, it wasn't achievement that saved her, but the steady presence of people who offered empathy, humor, and light.

- **David Foster Wallace** – Wallace's "This is Water" metaphor helped Elisa articulate the invisible forces that shape us—especially trauma we've never fully named. She used his image of fish asking, "What's water?" to convey how the death of her brother became the atmosphere of her life—so ever-present, she didn't know she was swimming in it until much later.

- **Benjamin Lee Whorf** – Before becoming a linguist, Whorf worked as an insurance assessor and noticed people were more reckless around "empty gasoline drums" than full ones—though the vapors were still dangerous. This led him to the Whorfian hypothesis: that language shapes perception. Sometimes, we can't even think a thought until we have the words to hold it. On the other hand, by choosing our words intentionally, we can shape our own thoughts.

- **Elie Wiesel** – Elisa quotes Wiesel's piercing response to the question "Where was God?"—his counter-question, *"Where was man?"* (from *Night*)—because it shifts the weight of meaning-making and moral responsibility onto humanity itself. Notably, Philip Yancey, writing from an evangelical Christian perspective, echoes this question in *Where Is God When It Hurts?*, asking instead, *"Where is the church?"* In the wake of immense suffering, it's tempting to direct our rage heavenward. But Wiesel, survivor of Auschwitz and tireless keeper of memory, urges us to look inward and outward—not merely upward—for accountability. His work invites us to reconsider the theology of suffering and to reclaim agency even in moments of devastation. His moral clarity and compassionate realism help anchor this memoir in something deeper than consolation—truth.

- **The Woman with the Alabaster Jar (John 12 / Mark 14)** – The woman who poured out a flask of pure nard—worth a year's wages—onto the feet of Jesus understood something most of us still struggle to grasp: that love and grief are often one and the same. In that sacred act of anointing, she wasn't just honoring him—she was preparing him. Her tears, her tenderness, her extravagance—they filled the room with the fragrance of what love looks like when it refuses to hold back. It was gratitude. It was mourning. It was worship. And it reminds us that sometimes the most meaningful goodbyes happen before the ending. Maybe this is the way they should be.

- **Philip Yancey** – In *Where Is God When It Hurts?*, Yancey writes not as someone with all the answers, but as a fellow traveler on the broken road. After exploring why physical pain is essential to our survival, he extends the metaphor to spiritual and emotional suffering, suggesting that pain also holds meaning in those realms. Rather than fixating on *why* pain exists, Yancey poses two deeper questions. First: *How will you respond to the pain?*—a question Elisa also invites readers to consider. Second: *Where is the church?*—a powerful echo of Elie Wiesel's haunting "Where was man?" Yancey directs this challenge specifically to the Christian community, urging them to be present in the face of suffering. His humility and reverence for mystery have helped many recognize that God is often found not in the thunder, but in the whisper. Elisa includes Yancey's work for those seeking a compassionate, evangelical Christian perspective on the problem of pain.

— · —

AUTHOR'S NOTE

DID THIS BOOK TOUCH YOU?

I f this book offered you comfort, courage, or companionship, would you consider leaving a few words behind—like a trail of light for someone else who might be searching? I'd be so blessed if you left a review on Amazon or Goodreads.

Thank you for carrying this story with you for a while.

Note on the Use of AI Assistance

Throughout the creation of this book, I used ChatGPT (a generative AI developed by OpenAI) as an editorial and research support tool which I call Hilda. I relied on Hilda's help to locate and format sources in MLA style, synthesize and summarize research from books I personally read, and identify new titles to further my study. I used it to check each paragraph for coherence, accuracy, grammar, and clarity—especially when I needed help untangling dense or emotionally charged material. I also used it to help me assess tone, striving to ensure that my words would not unintentionally harm or alienate anyone.

ChatGPT generated early drafts of discussion questions and Notes on Quotes, which I then culled, reshaped, or rewrote entirely. On occasion, I asked it to help rework a paragraph that wasn't quite expressing what I meant.

All of the content, ideas, reflections, and stories in this book are wholly my own. ChatGPT did not originate anything in these pages—it simply helped me say what I meant to say, more clearly and more compassionately.

— • —

ACKNOWLEDGEMENTS

First, my undying gratitude to Brian and Diane, who through their lives and deaths and our relationships, have largely defined me. You are always with me, in every cell of my being and your light flickers on every page I write. And to my mother, my comrade in grief. Your legendary strength has always been the gold standard to which I aspire. I wouldn't have been able to achieve a single thing without your loving sacrifices. And to the memory of my father, who took such delight in warping—I mean, shaping my mind. I know he is proud beyond the grave. Thank you also to my sister, Loi, for being loyal above all else. And loving gratitude to the memory of my brother Eric, the funniest man I knew. I hope he would have chuckled throughout this book.

To my chosen bonus family of to-the-death friends, Lena, Mike, Tina, Dee, Maranda, and John, thank you for being such an important part of my resurrection. Thank you also for such extraordinary care for me in my illness during covid. Several of you isolated yourselves for me for many months, and I don't have words to thank you for your sacrifices. You kept me alive in body, mind, and hilarity. You cooked, you cried, you carried me (literally), and you cussed creatively on my behalf. Even death will not us part. To my adoptive daughters, Malalai and Zarmina, I can't believe God blessed me with you. I want to be like you when I grow up. To Asnah, you are the little girl I always dreamed of having. I love you more than life. To my medical team at NIH, a secret city of angels tucked away in Bethesda, I wouldn't be alive without you. Every time I came to NIH it was a joy, no matter what the circumstances, sick as I was. Thank you for being both brilliant and human. To my nurses, especially Dianna, Amanda, Ola, and Kaya, you were so wonderful you absolutely gave me something to look forward to in coming in for chemo. Dianna, I'll never forget how you held my hand at the hospital during covid when my blood pressure had been 63/33 and my heart rate was in the 160s.

To the readers of my blog, friends, family and students, you gave me purpose and kept me engaged and full of hope throughout my illness. You inspired me to pour out my soul and ultimately to write this book. To Karen Snyder, you are so good at lifting others up; you have been a mentor and a major inspiration to me.

To my editor, Katrina Schroeder, and to Amy M. Le: Thank you for helping me make this dream a reality.

To my beta reader, Tamara Dragseth, thank you for such thoughtful and helpful feedback. I reshaped my manuscript in response, and it is a far better book for it.

To Lena Monje, Mike Croghan, Soncee Brown, Audrey Anthony, Kate Maisel, Pat Monahan, Rachel Creager, Robin Patrick, Annette Cowart, Maren Tirabassi, Ann Murdoch, Deanna D'Arcy, and Alice Marks — thank you for loving me enough to read drafts of my book and offer your generous, loving feedback.

To Maren especially — thank you for the wisdom you've shared as someone who has written more than twenty beautiful books yourself.

To the friends who came back to me and were right there loving me throughout my cancer even though our connection was remote, Soncee, Robin, Hiroko, Angela, Anna, Rachel, Allison, Terri, and Hannah, cancer was absolutely a fair price to pay to have you close again. To the poets, mystics, theologians and other bright souls who lit the way, how would I shine if you had not shined your light on me? To Daniel Jones (pseudonym), the psychiatrist who specialized in early childhood grief and guided me through trauma therapy — you are so much the reason for my resurrection. I love you.

To my past self: Congratulations. You lived to be less than half a pencil, and I trust you'll have enough left to write all the books already inscribed in your soul.

To my present self: Enjoy this delicious life you have.

To my future self: Surprise me.

And finally, to the Spirit of Life Herself, I am so happy to be full of light, full of love, full of joy and full of You.

ABOUT THE AUTHOR

Elisa L. Everts is a writer, professor of ESL, and grief educator (currently pursuing an MA in Thanatology) with a Ph.D. in sociolinguistics from Georgetown University and a passion for language as a tool for healing. A Stage IV cancer survivor, lifelong teacher, and adoptive mother of many, she writes at the intersection of grief, storytelling, spirituality, and joy. Her work is rooted in the belief that suffering can be a sacred space—and that even the shadow of death is not black, but technicolor.

She has spent over three decades teaching ESL, culture, linguistics, and the power of words in the U.S., Japan, and Korea. She always says, *I study language because I want to learn how we can use language to love people better.* Her academic writing has appeared in the peer-reviewed journal the *International Journal of Humor Research*, (John Benjamins) and the edited volume, *Discourse and Technology* (Georgetown University Press), where she explored the intersections of identity, narrative, blind/sighted interaction, humor, and family discourse. Her poetry has been published in various journals.

When she's not writing books or guiding field trips to museums with adult ESL students, she's reaching out to new Afghan refugees, working on a graduate degree in Thanatology, writing long-ass emails to loved ones, or searching for metaphors sharp enough to cut through denial.

Elisa lives in Virginia next door to her Afghan family (Malalai, Edris, Asnah, Zaki and Foroogh), with two adorable rescue cats named Maxine and Rafiki, and more poetry anthologies than strictly necessary. *I Should Wake Before I Die* is her debut memoir. She is currently polishing her next book—*Gasping for Light*, a collection of reflections, poetry and prayers to feed the grieving soul. Designed to be a companion in life's hardest seasons—whether you're undergoing treatment, grieving a loss, or simply searching for light—it offers comfort, courage, and moments of meaning when you need them most.

Say hello or follow her writing at and on Instagram **@Elisa_L_Everts.**

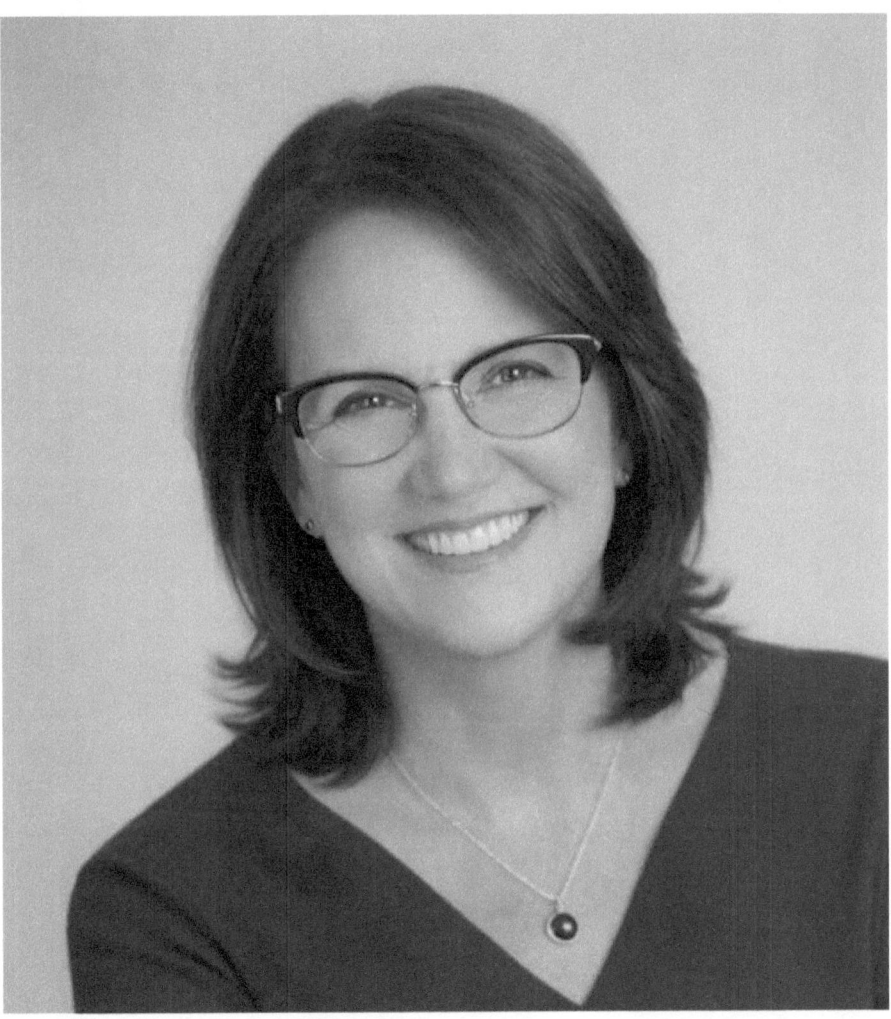